COLOUR GUIDE

# Surgical Pathology

**W. E. G. Thomas** BSc MBBS FRCS MS
Consultant Surgeon, Royal Hallamshire Hospital,
Sheffield; Court of Examiners and Hunterian Professor,
Royal College of Surgeons; Moynihan Fellow,
Association of Surgeons

**J. H. F. Smith** BSc MBBS MRCPath
Consultant Histopathologist, Northern General
Hospital, Sheffield; Honorary Clinical Lecturer,
University of Sheffield

Churchill Livingstone

EDINBURGH LONDON MADRID MELBOURNE NEW

# Preface

The aim of this book is to provide senior undergraduates and surgical
postgraduates with a pictorial guide to surgical pathology. By including both
macroscopical and microscopical illustrations of common surgical
conditions, it is hoped that it will prove of particular value to those
candidates sitting the FRCS examination. It will also be of value to trainee
pathologists, enabling them to recognize classical pathology patterns. It is
not a pathological textbook, but seeks to introduce each subject in as concise
a manner as possible.

We are extremely grateful to many of our colleagues for assisting us in
assembling this collection of illustrations, and to our publishers who have
patiently and graciously waited while the collection has been compiled.

Sheffield                                                        W.E.G.T.
1992                                                             J.H.F.S.

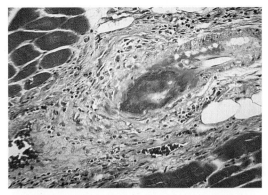

**Fig. 1** Polyarteritis nodosa. Fibrinoid necrosis and inflammation of vessel wall. MSB × 10.

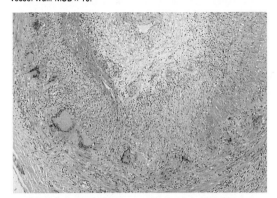

**Fig. 2** Giant cell arteritis. Note giant cells, intimal thickening and inflammation.

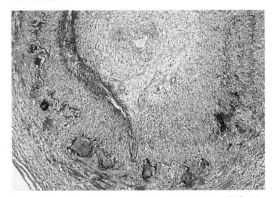

**Fig. 3** Giant cell arteritis. Fragmentation of elastic lamina. EVG ×25.

# 2 / Blood vessels: aneurysms

*Definition*  A localized dilatation of an artery. True aneurysms result from stretching of vessel wall. False aneurysms result from perforation of the vessel wall and are bound by connective tissue.

## Atheromatous aneurysms

*Incidence*  Usually men over the age of 50 yrs.

*Aetiology*  Associated with severe atheroma.

*Site*  May affect any artery, but typically the abdominal aorta, iliac, femoral and popliteal arteries.

*Macroscopical*  Fusiform (Fig. 4) or saccular dilatation of the vessel, often partially occluded by thrombus.

*Microscopical*  Pressure atrophy or destruction of the media by extensive severe atheromatous plaques (Fig. 5).

*Effects*  ● Rupture and haemorrhage.
● Distal ischaemia from thrombosis or embolism.
● Pulsatile mass with pressure symptoms.

## Syphilitic aneurysms

*Incidence*  Now rare. Usually over the age of 40 yrs.

*Aetiology*  Syphilitic aortitis weakening the aortic wall.

*Site*  Usually ascending or transverse arch of aorta.

*Macroscopical*  Saccular aneurysm (Fig. 6) with intimal scarring.

*Microscopical*  Adventitial vessels show perivascular plasma cell and lymphocytic infiltrate with ischaemic atrophy of medial elastic tissue and smooth muscle, and replacement by fibrous tissue.

*Effects*  Pressure symptoms, rupture, aortic incompetence due to valve ring involvement, thrombosis and embolism.

# Contents

# 1 / Blood vessels: the vasculitides

*Introduction*  Arteritis, vasculitis and angiitis are terms to describe inflammation of arteries, veins and capillaries respectively. Inflammation may result from direct damage (e.g. trauma, toxins, irradiation), but the most important are the 'non-infective necrotizing vasculitides'.

## Polyarteritis nodosa

*Nature*  A disease of small or medium-sized arteries, usually involving renal and other visceral vessels.

*Incidence*  Young adults — M:F = 2–3:1.

*Macroscopical*  Scattered visceral infarcts of varying ages.

*Microscopical*  In acute lesions (Fig. 1) there is fibrinoid necrosis of the vessel wall with transmural neutrophil infiltrate and often thrombosis. Healing lesions show mural fibroblastic proliferation with microaneurysm formation.

*Prognosis*  60–80% 5 yr survival. Death occurs from renal failure and visceral haemorrhage or infarction.

## Giant cell (temporal) arteritis

*Nature*  Focal granulomatous inflammation of muscular arteries affecting mainly cranial vessels.

*Incidence*  Rare under 50 yrs. Women more than men.

*Macroscopical*  Tenderness and erythema over temporal artery. Widespread visceral infarction may occur in systemic disease. Visual symptoms are common.

*Microscopical*  Non-specific inflammatory infiltrate, intimal fibrosis and multinucleate giant cells related to degenerate internal elastic lamina (Figs 2 & 3).

*Prognosis*  Excellent response to steroids. Rarely, widespread systemic involvement may be fatal.

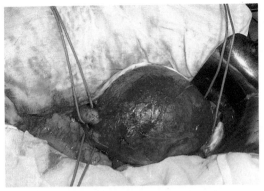

**Fig. 4** Fusiform atheromatous aneurysm of the abdominal aorta.

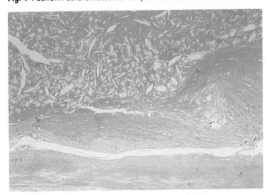

**Fig. 5** Atheromatous plaque in the wall of an aneurysm.

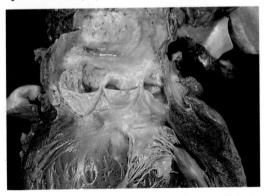

**Fig. 6** Syphilitic aneurysm. Note dilatation of aortic root and intimal roughening.

## Dissecting aneurysm

*Definition*   Splitting of the wall of an artery, so that blood tracks along the media in a false lumen.

*Incidence*   Most common in hypertensive males over 40 yrs.

*Aetiology*   Unknown, but most are associated with cystic medial necrosis (Erdheim's mucoid degeneration).

*Site*   The aorta.

*Macroscopical*   There is a transverse intimal tear (Fig. 7) in the ascending aortic arch, with blood tracking into the media and extending in both directions.

*Microscopical*   Focal separation of elastic and fibromuscular elements of the media (Fig. 8) by clefts filled with mucoid material (cystic medial necrosis). Fragmentation of the elastic laminae and haemorrhage in the media.

*Effects*
- Re-entry into lumen—double-barrelled aorta.
- Rupture into pericardium, pleura, peritoneum.
- Occlusion of aortic side branches, e.g. coronary, renal, mesenteric arteries.
- Aortic incompetence, dilatation of valve ring.

## Congenital aneurysms — berry aneurysms

*Incidence*   Commonest cause of subarachnoid haemorrhage.

*Aetiology*   Congenital defect of media at vessel junctions.

*Macroscopical*   Solitary or multiple berry-like aneurysms found on the circle of Willis and its branches (Fig. 9).

*Microscopical*   Fibrous walled vessel without media.

*Effects*   Rupture produces subarachnoid haemorrhage. 25–60% die with the first bleed. It occasionally presents with pressure effects or intracerebral haemorrhage.

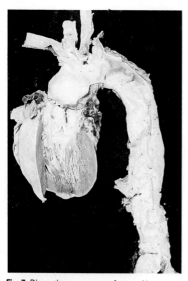

**Fig. 7** Dissecting aneurysm of aorta. Note transverse intimal tear.

**Fig. 8** Aortic medionecrosis. Deposits of myxoid substance within vessel media. H&E ×25.

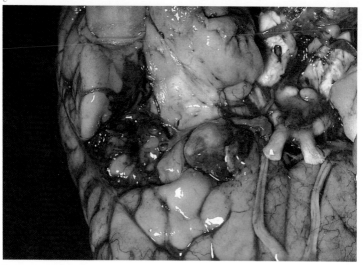

**Fig. 9** Ruptured berry aneurysm of anterior communicating cerebral artery.

# 3 / Tuberculosis (TB)

| | |
|---|---|
| *Definition* | A chronic bacterial granulomatous infection caused by *Mycobacterium tuberculosis*. |
| *Incidence* | Diminishing in incidence (now approximately 500 deaths/yr, 9000 new cases/yr). It is seen mainly in immigrants or the elderly, representing recrudescence of healed primary or secondary lesions associated with silicosis, immunosuppression, alcohol or diabetes mellitus. |

## Primary pulmonary tuberculosis

| | |
|---|---|
| *Macroscopical* | A single mid-zone subpleural yellow nodule (Ghon focus), with marked enlargement and caseous necrosis of tracheobronchial and mediastinal lymph nodes (primary complex) (Fig. 10). |
| *Microscopical* | Granulomas composed of a central area of eosinophilic caseous necrosis surrounded by epithelioid macrophages, lymphocytes and multinucleate Langhans giant cells (Fig. 12). |
| *Prognosis* | Progressive healing with fibrosis is usual, but direct spread to pleura and adjacent lung, blood-borne spread to single organs or widespread dissemination (miliary TB) may occur. |

## Secondary pulmonary tuberculosis

| | |
|---|---|
| *Macroscopical* | Caseous necrosis with cavitation in the apical lung segments. Hilar nodes rarely affected. |

## Miliary tuberculosis

| | |
|---|---|
| *Aetiology* | Tuberculous bacteraemia giving rise to numerous tubercles in various organs, especially lung. |
| *Macroscopical* | The lung is studded with numerous pale grey tubercles up to a few millimetres in diameter (Fig. 11). |
| *Prognosis* | Untreated miliary TB is rapidly fatal. |

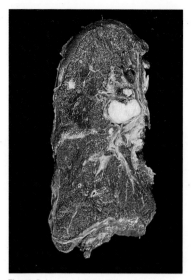

**Fig. 10** Pulmonary tuberculosis: primary complex.

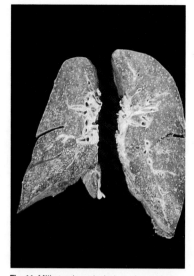

**Fig. 11** Miliary tuberculosis. Lung is studded with numerous grey tubercles.

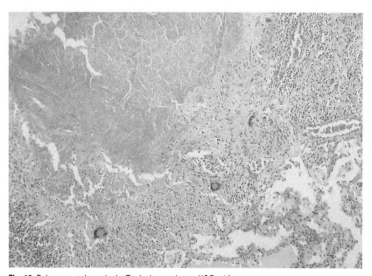

**Fig. 12** Pulmonary tuberculosis. Typical granuloma. H&E ×10.

# 4 / Tumours of the lungs

## Adenochondroma (hamartomatous chondroma)

Definition : Rare abnormal mixture of pulmonary components.

Aetiology : Probably an overgrowth of bronchial wall mesenchymal components with secondary entrapment of bronchial epithelium.

Macroscopical : Subpleural, well-defined, lobulated, blue/grey mass composed largely of cartilage (Fig. 13). Often incidental radiological finding.

Microscopical : Nodules of cartilage, associated with fibrous and adipose tissue and bronchial epithelium (Fig. 14). Calcification and ossification may occur.

Prognosis : Excision excludes malignancy and is curative.

## Benign tumours

Benign epithelial tumours (adenomas, papillomas) and soft tissue tumours (lipomas, leiomyomas) occur in bronchi and lung but are all rare.

## Carcinoid tumours

Definition : Tumour of bronchial argentaffin cells.

Incidence : About 5% of all bronchial neoplasms. M:F = 1:1.

Macroscopical : Vascular grey/yellow endobronchial tumour.

Microscopical : Mosaic or trabecular pattern of polygonal cells with granular eosinophilic or clear cytoplasm, regular oval nuclei and prominent nucleoli but few mitoses. Majority show positive argyrophil staining (Fig. 15) with dense core granules on electron microscopy.

Prognosis : Low grade malignant tumour, slow growing with potential to metastasise to regional nodes. If disseminated, occasionally produces the carcinoid syndrome.

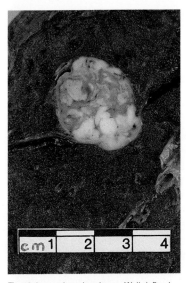

**Fig. 13** Lung adenochondroma. Well-defined solid lesion with variegated cut surface.

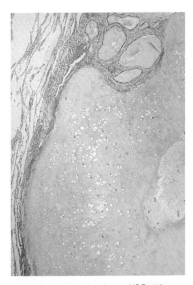

**Fig. 14** Lung adenochondroma. H&E ×10.

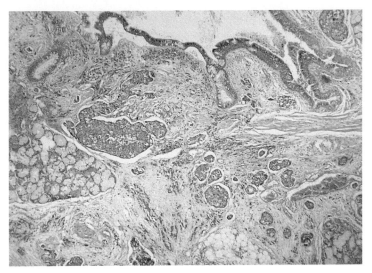

**Fig. 15** Bronchial carcinoid tumour. Multiple nests and islands of uniform round cells. H&E ×10.

## Carcinoma

*Definition*    Malignant epithelial tumour arising in bronchi or lung parenchyma.

*Incidence*    In England and Wales, the largest cause of cancer deaths in men (26 000 deaths/yr) and third largest in women (9000 deaths/yr).

*Aetiology*    Cigarette smoking is the most important factor; others recognized are asbestos, cobalt and chromate exposure, nickel refining and haematite mining.

*Macroscopical*    A firm grey/white mass, usually arising close to origin of main lobar bronchi, presenting either as a stenotic ulcerating mass, an infiltrating peribronchial mass or a cauliflower like intraparenchymal tumour growing from the bronchus (Fig. 16). A few (mainly adenocarcinomas) arise peripherally and are often associated with areas of scarring (Fig. 17); one variant (bronchioloalveolar) grows along alveolar walls with mucin secretion producing a mucoid grey cut surface.

*Microscopical*    Four principal histological types are recognized.

*Squamous cell carcinoma.* (Fig. 18). Composed of malignant epithelial cells showing keratinization, with keratin pearl formation and/or intercellular bridges.

*Small cell carcinoma.* Composed of loosely aggregated round or oval cells about twice the size of lymphocytes with scanty indistinct cytoplasm (oat cell carcinoma) (Fig. 19). Spindle and polygonal varieties are also recognized. Usually centrally located, and widely disseminated when diagnosed, the primary tumour is often small and inconspicuous, but may produce systemic effects from inappropriate hormone production.

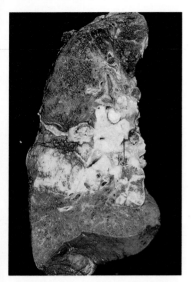

**Fig. 16** Primary bronchial carcinoma situated at pulmonary hilum.

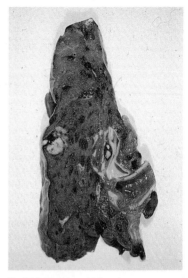

**Fig. 17** Primary bronchial carcinoma at periphery of lung.

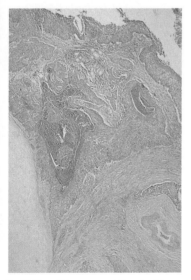

**Fig. 18** Bronchial squamous cell carcinoma. Note abundant keratin formation. H&E ×10.

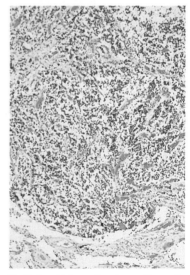

**Fig. 19** Bronchial oat cell carcinoma. Sheets of undifferentiated hyperchromatic cells. H&E ×25.

*Microscopical*    **Adenocarcinoma.** Takes two forms, either acinar adenocarcinoma with a predominance of glandular structures, or bronchioloalveolar carcinoma in which the cylindrical malignant epithelial cells grow on the walls of pre-existing alveoli (Fig. 20). Both principal types produce variable amounts of mucin.

**Large cell carcinoma.** (Fig. 21). Composed of large polygonal cells with vesicular nuclei, well defined cell bodies and frequent mitoses. Some subtypes are composed mainly of clear cells (clear cell carcinoma), or bizarre multinucleate giant cells (giant cell carcinoma). Electron microscopy shows that some are undifferentiated squamous or adenocarcinomas. They are usually centrally located.

*Prognosis*    Surgical resection offers the best hope of cure, but the majority are inoperable. Overall outlook is poor, 10% 5 yr survival for squamous and adenocarcinomas, but only 3% for small and large cell carcinomas. For widely disseminated tumours, chemotherapy/radiotherapy is utilized.

## Secondary tumours

The lung is a frequent site for secondary metastases from sarcomas and carcinomas by blood-borne, lymphatic or direct spread.

*Macroscopical*    Either multiple discrete nodules (Fig. 22), diffuse tumour infiltrates in peribronchiolar and perivesicular tissue spaces, or diffuse permeation of subpleural lymphatics (lymphangitis carcinomatosa). Sarcomas usually present as multiple nodules while carcinomas present in all three forms.

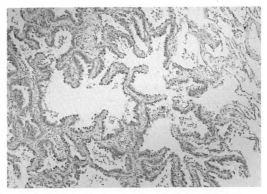

**Fig. 20** Bronchioloalveolar cell carcinoma. Typical lepidic growth pattern. H&E ×25.

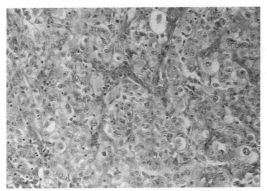

**Fig. 21** Large cell anaplastic carcinoma of the lung. H&E ×25.

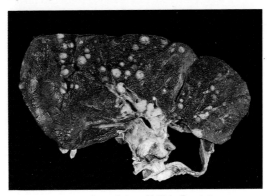

**Fig. 22** Metastatic carcinoma in lung. Multiple discrete tumour deposits in lung parenchyma.

# 5 / **Lymph nodes: reactive disorders**

*Definition*    Lymph nodes respond rapidly to the presence of local inflammation or foreign material, and this process is known as reactive hyperplasia. It presents in one of three microscopical forms depending on the nature of the provoking agent.

*Aetiology*    Many agents produce non-specific changes, but others can produce typical patterns that are of diagnostic value, e.g. toxoplasmosis, cat scratch disease. Other disease processes produce chronic specific granulomatous change, e.g. tuberculosis, sarcoid, syphilis.

*Macroscopical*    Affected nodes are enlarged, soft and fleshy. It is often not possible to distinguish from neoplastic lymphadenopathy.

*Microscopical*    **Paracortical hyperplasia** (Fig. 23). Follows a cell-mediated response and is characterized by enlargement of the 'T-cell' dependent, paracortical (parafollicular) zone.

**Follicular hyperplasia** (Fig. 24). Follows a humoral response mediated by 'B' lymphocytes and is characterized by hyperplastic cortical follicles and germinal centres.

**Sinus hyperplasia** (Fig. 25). Follows exposure to foreign materials which evoke intense phagocytic activity, leading to hyperplasia and enlargement of the phagocytic sinus-lining cells.

*Prognosis*    Depends on the precipitating cause. In many cases, once the provoking agent is removed, the hyperplasia resolves. For infective causes, specific therapy may lead to resolution.

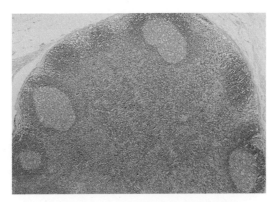

**Fig. 23** Lymph node: reactive paracortical hyperplasia. H&E.

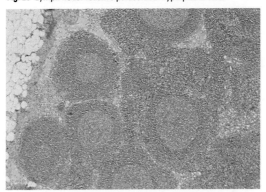

**Fig. 24** Lymph node: reactive follicular hyperplasia. H&E.

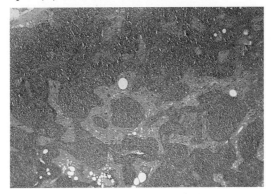

**Fig. 25** Lymph node: reactive sinus histiocytosis. H&E.

# 6 / Lymph nodes: malignant disorders

*Definition*  Lymph node malignancy consists of neoplastic proliferation of lymphoid cell lines (malignant lymphoma) or metastatic deposits. Malignant lymphoma is divided into two broad groups.

## Hodgkin's disease (HD)

*Incidence*  HD is the most common malignant lymphoma.

*Macroscopical*  Rubbery enlargement of lymph nodes.

*Microscopical*  Destruction of nodal architecture and replacement by a mixture of lymphocytes, eosinophils and plasma cells with large, pale staining, histiocyte-like cells. Some of these are multinucleate or binucleate, with prominent nucleoli and a 'mirror-image' configuration (Fig. 26). These Reed-Sternberg cells are essential for the diagnosis of HD.

## Non-hodgkin's lymphoma (NHL)

The diversity of different classifications and terminologies reflects current uncertainty as to the histiogenesis of many subtypes of NHL.

*Microscopical*  Classification is based on two factors:
- Growth pattern—follicular or diffuse.
- Constituent cell type, i.e. T- or B-cell lymphocytes, follicle centre cells (centrocytes and centroblasts), histiocytes or plasma cells.

In general, follicular NHL (Fig. 27) has a reasonable prognosis, while diffuse NHL has a poor prognosis (Fig. 28).

## Metastatic tumour

Lymph nodes are a frequent site for metastatic tumour, especially carcinoma. Nodal involvement usually starts in the subcapsular sinus and spreads to replace the rest of the node.

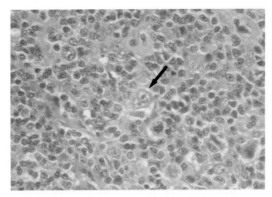

**Fig. 26** Lymph node: Hodgkin's disease. H&E ×25. Characteristic Reed-Sternberg cell (arrowed).

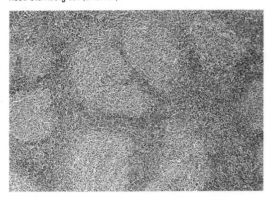

**Fig. 27** Lymph node: follicular non-Hodgkin's lymphoma (compare with Fig. 24). H&E ×10.

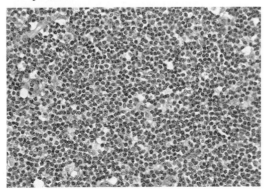

**Fig. 28** Diffuse lymphocytic non-Hodgkin's lymphoma. H&E ×25.

# 7 / **Salivary glands**

## Sjögren's syndrome

*Definition*    Autoimmune destruction of salivary and lacrimal glands (sicca syndrome; dry eyes and mouth).

*Aetiology*    60–80% have antibodies to nuclear antigens.

*Microscopical*    Destructive lymphocytic and plasma cell infiltration of gland parenchyma (Fig. 29).

*Outcome*    Increased risk of lymphoid malignancy.

## Pleomorphic adenoma

*Incidence*    50–75% of all parotid tumours. M:F = 1:3.

*Nature*    Arises from epithelial and myoepithelial cells.

*Macroscopical*    Encapsulated, lobulated mass with fleshy cut surface containing blue-grey mucoid areas.

*Microscopical*    Heterogenous mixture of epithelial cells (ducts, acini, tubules, microcysts), myoepithelial elements (small, dark, polygonal cells) and mesenchymal elements (myxoid stroma with cartilaginous or osseous differentiation) (Fig. 30).

*Prognosis*    5–50% recur from residual pseudopodia after enucleation. The tumours rarely become malignant.

## Adenolymphoma (Warthin's tumour)

*Incidence*    5–15% of parotid tumours. Usually occurs in elderly men.

*Nature*    Epithelial origin and reactive lymphoid element.

*Macroscopical*    Soft encapsulated mass with visible clefts or cysts containing cloudy fluid.

*Microscopical*    Cystic glandular spaces lined by double-layered columnar epithelium over lymphoid tissue (Fig. 31).

*Prognosis*    Benign. Rarely recurs.

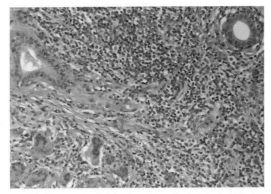

**Fig. 29** Salivary gland: Sjögren's syndrome. Typical lymphoepithelial lesion. H&E.

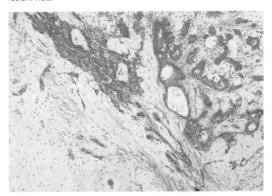

**Fig. 30** Salivary gland: pleomorphic adenoma. H&E.

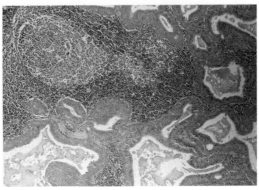

**Fig. 31** Salivary gland: adenolymphoma. H&E.

## Mucoepidermoid tumour

*Incidence*  2–7% of salivary tumours; usually in the parotid.

*Macroscopical*  Poorly defined, partially encapsulated, solid cystic or semi-cystic tumour.

*Microscopical*  Cords, sheets or cystic configurations of squamous and mucus-secreting cells (Fig. 32).

*Prognosis*  Unpredictable, but poor if histological evidence of lymphatic invasion or capsule infiltration.

## Acinic cell tumour

*Incidence*  Uncommon; 1–3% of parotid tumours.

*Nature*  Possibly arises from multipotential duct cells.

*Macroscopical*  Encapsulated lobulated tumour with areas of necrosis and haemorrhage.

*Microscopical*  Cords, sheets or glandular arrangements of rounded cells similar to normal acinar cells (Fig. 33).

*Prognosis*  75% 5 yr survival after adequate resection.

## Adenoid cystic carcinoma (cylindroma)

*Incidence*  Most common malignancy in minor salivary glands, accounting for 2–3% of parotid and 11–17% of submandibular tumours.

*Aetiology*  Derived from duct or myoepithelial cells.

*Macroscopical*  Infiltrative firm grey-white tumour.

*Microscopical*  Tubular, solid or cribriform arrangement of cells enclosing cystic spaces (Fig. 34).

*Prognosis*  Poor. Aggressive local perineural infiltration and lymphatic metastases.

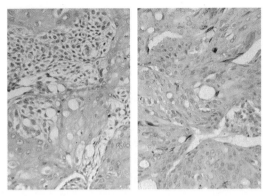

**Fig. 32** Mucoepidermoid carcinoma. Note squamous and glandular differentiation H&E ×25 (left), AB/PAS (right).

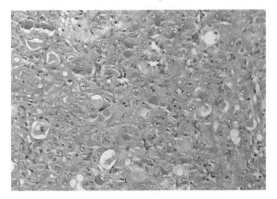

**Fig. 33** Salivary gland: acinic cell tumour. H&E ×25.

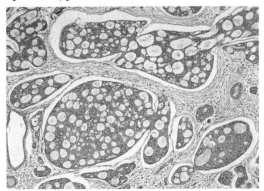

**Fig. 34** Salivary gland: adenoid cystic carcinoma (cylindroma). H&E ×25.

# 8 / **Oesophagus**

## Inflammation

Opportunistic infections, e.g. candidiasis, may occur with reduced immunity. Gastric reflux may cause peptic oesophagitis, and the lower oesophagus can become lined by metaplastic columnar epithelium (Barrett's oesophagus).

## Circulatory disorders

Submucosal veins in the lower oesophagus are a site of portosystemic anastomosis. In portal hypertension they become distended to form varices (Fig. 35): fatal haemorrhage can occur.

## Tumours

Benign tumours are rare. Leiomyoma is the commonest, presenting as an intraluminal polyp.

### Carcinoma

*Incidence* — Commonest oesophageal tumour. M:F = 5:1.

*Aetiology* — Unknown. There is marked geographical variation. It is common in Iran, North China and the Transkei. Pre-existing oesophageal disease may predispose, e.g. oesophagitis, achalasia, diverticula, webs, Barrett's oesophagus. Irritants such as spicy foods, alcohol and smoking are also implicated.

*Macroscopical* — Polypoid fungating (Fig. 36), ulcerating or diffusely infiltrative lesion with submucosal spread and involvement of local structures.

*Microscopical* — Majority are squamous carcinomas (Fig. 37). In the lower oesophagus some are adenocarcinomas spreading upwards from the stomach, or arising from Barrett's oesophagus. Mucoepidermoid, adenoid cystic and primary oat cell carcinomas of the oesophagus have also been described.

*Prognosis* — Resection possible in less than 50%. Overall, 70% die within 1 yr, with 5–10% 5 yr survival.

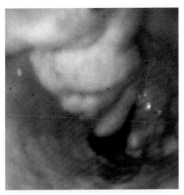

**Fig. 35** Endoscopic view of oesophageal varices.

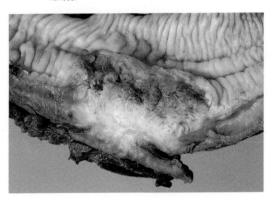

**Fig. 36** Oesophagus: longitudinal section to show ulcerated carcinoma.

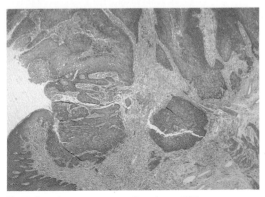

**Fig. 37** Oesophagus: squamous cell carcinoma. H&E.

# 9 / **Pyloric stenosis and gastritis**

## Congenital hypertrophic pyloric stenosis

*Incidence*  Presents 2–6 wks after birth in 1 in 300–900 live births; M:F = 6:1. Increased incidence in siblings.

*Aetiology*  Unknown. Pyloric muscular hypertrophy leads to gastric outlet obstruction and projectile vomiting. Increased incidence in siblings suggests genetic predisposition.

*Macroscopical*  Greatly hypertrophied circular muscle fibres at pylorus presenting as pyloric 'tumour' (Fig. 38).

*Microscopical*  Smooth muscle hypertrophy.

*Prognosis*  Excellent following pyloromyotomy (Ramstedt's procedure).

## Acute gastritis

*Definition*  Acute inflammation of gastric mucosa, usually of transient nature.

*Aetiology*  Frequently associated with excess alcohol, heavy smoking, chronic aspirin ingestion, certain chemotherapeutic agents, uraemia, systemic infection (especially in children) and stress, i.e. burns, shock, irradiation. It may result from gastric mucosal barrier damage allowing $H^+$ ion back diffusion and/or mucosal hypoperfusion.

*Macroscopical*  Varies from moderate oedema and slight hyperaemia to extensive sloughing with haemorrhage (erosions) (Fig. 39).

*Microscopical*  Variable oedema and congestion of the lamina propria with an infiltrate of polymorphonuclear leucocytes (Fig. 40).

*Prognosis*  Severe gastritis can lead to haematemesis and melaena. Healing usually follows removal of the insulting agent.

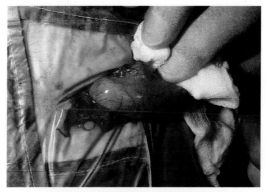

**Fig. 38** The 'tumour' of infantile hypertrophic pyloric stenosis.

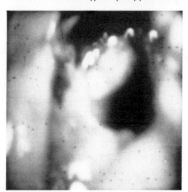

**Fig. 39** Endoscopic view of acute erosive gastritis.

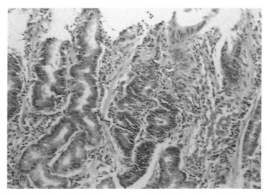

**Fig. 40** Acute gastritis. Note polymorph infiltrate and superficial ulceration. H&E.

## Diffuse chronic gastritis (type A)

*Aetiology*    Possibly autoimmune. May have parietal cell and intrinsic factor antibodies, and suffer from pernicious anaemia, diabetes, hypoadrenalism, Hashimoto's disease and hypoparathyroidism.

*Distribution*    Affects acid secreting mucosa of body/fundus.

*Macroscopical*    Superficial chronic gastritis is not visually recognizable; atrophic gastritis shows mucosal flattening and loss of rugae. In gastric atrophy there is marked mucosal thinning.

*Microscopical*    **Superficial chronic gastritis:** (Fig. 41) increased gastric pit length, with lymphocyte and plasma cell infiltrate in the lamina propria.

**Atrophic gastritis:** (Fig. 42) similar changes, with loss of parietal and chief cells being replaced by mucous epithelium (pseudopyloric metaplasia), or goblet, Paneth and absorptive cells (intestinal metaplasia).

**Gastric atrophy:** (Fig. 43) diffuse mucosal atrophy, virtually complete pseudopyloric and intestinal metaplasia and lamina propria oedema.

*Effects*    Hypochlorhydria progressing to achlorhydria.

## Multifocal chronic gastritis (type B)

*Aetiology*    Not immunological. Bile reflux, alcohol, tobacco, hot fluids and salicylates are all implicated.

*Distribution*    Patchy involvement of junction between body and antrum. Later becomes confluent.

*Macroscopical*    As above.

*Microscopical*    As above but more active inflammation in pits.

*Effects*    May cause dyspepsia. Possibly predisposes to peptic ulcer and even gastric carcinoma.

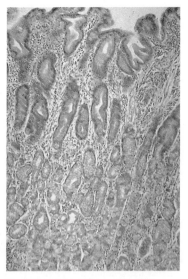

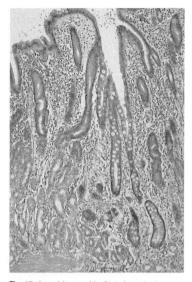

**Fig. 41** Superficial chronic gastritis. H&E.

**Fig. 42** Atrophic gastritis. Note intestinal metaplasia. H&E.

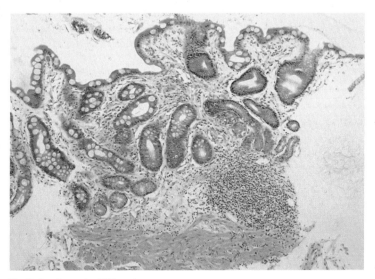

**Fig. 43** Gastric atrophy. H&E.

# 10 / **Peptic ulceration**

*Definition*  A breach of surface epithelium by an interaction of acid and pepsin on the mucosa.

## Gastric ulcer

*Incidence*  Regional variation. More common in men, the elderly, lower socioeconomic groups and blood group A.

*Aetiology*  Unknown. Damage to mucosal barrier can allow back diffusion of $H^+$ ions, resulting in mucosal damage, e.g. duodenogastric reflux, antral stasis, alcohol, salicylates, non-steroidal anti-inflammatory agents or corticosteroids.

*Macroscopical*  *Acute:* often multiple superficial erosions.
*Chronic:* (Fig. 44) deep ulcers with fibrotic base usually at junction of fundic and antral mucosa. Raised or indurated edges may suggest malignancy.

*Microscopical*  Fibrinous exudate covering granulation tissue over dense fibrotic base, occupying full thickness defect in muscularis (Fig. 45).

*Effects*  High incidence of recurrence. May perforate, bleed or cause stenosis and outlet obstruction. The risk of malignant change is undefined.

## Duodenal ulcer

*Incidence*  Declining, particularly in relation to male prevalence, perforation and mortality.

*Aetiology*  Controversial. Parietal cell hyperplasia due to increased vagal activity, decreased inhibition of secretion and, occasionally, hypergastrinaemia (Zollinger-Ellison syndrome) may produce acid hypersecretion and mucosal damage. Associated with smoking, stress, cirrhosis and blood group O.

*Effects*  May bleed, perforate or cause pyloric /duodenal stenosis. No increased risk of malignancy.

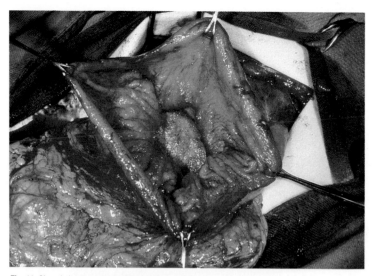

**Fig. 44** Chronic benign gastric ulcer.

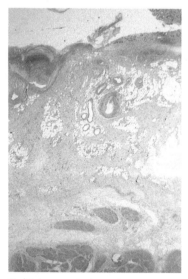

**Fig. 45** Acute peptic ulcer with haemorrhage. Note vessel in ulcer base. H&E ×2.5

# 11 / Tumours of the stomach

## Benign tumours

These comprise of *leiomyomas*, which can ulcerate and haemorrhage, and *polyps*, which are regenerative (inflammatory, 80%), adenomatous (20%) and hamartomatous (1%). Adenomas carry a risk of malignant change.

## Malignant tumours

Lymphoma and soft tissue sarcomas are seen, but carcinoma predominates clinically.

### Carcinoma

*Incidence*    Highest in Japan, Chile, Iceland and Finland where mortality is 5–6 times that of USA and UK.

*Aetiology*    Unknown, but diet, cooking methods, socio-economic status and genetic factors of family history and blood group A may contribute; there is an increased risk with chronic atrophic gastritis (pernicious anaemia) and gastric adenomas.

*Macroscopical*    Majority occur in pylorus and antrum (60%). May be fungating (Fig. 46), ulcerated, infiltrative, polypoid or diffusely infiltrative (linitis plastica) (Fig. 47).

*Microscopical*    • Intestinal type with glandular pattern of pleomorphic cells and scanty mucin (Fig. 48). Occur in high risk areas and the elderly and are usually well defined.
  • Diffuse type of small uniform cells with plentiful mucin but few glandular lumina (Fig. 49). Usually the infiltrative form (linitis plastica).

*Prognosis*    Depends on clinical staging and lymph node involvement. There is a 30% 5 yr survival with no node involvement, but this falls to 5–10% with nodal metastases.

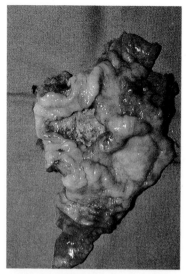

**Fig. 46** Ulcerated fungating carcinoma of the stomach.

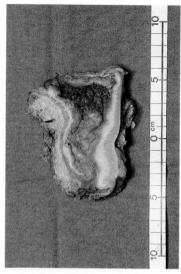

**Fig. 47** Linitis plastica of the stomach.

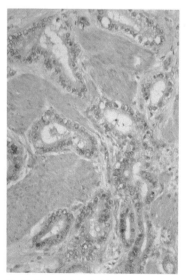

**Fig. 48** Stomach: intestinal type of adenocarcinoma. H&E ×64.

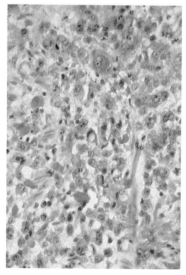

**Fig. 49** Diffuse infiltrative type of gastric adenocarcinoma. Note signet ring cells. H&E ×64.

# 12 / Ischaemic bowel

*Definition*   Hypoxic damage to bowel resulting from vascular compromise from occlusion or hypotension.

*Aetiology*   Vascular occlusion usually follows arterial embolism or thrombosis, but may occur with venous thrombosis, dissecting aneurysms, trauma, strangulation, arteritis or complications of angiography or neoplasia. Splanchnic hypotension occurs in cardiac failure or shock of any cause. Such hypotension superimposed on incomplete occlusion can result in ischaemia.

*Macroscopical*   Depends on nature, extent and duration of ischaemia. Infarcted bowel (Fig. 50) is initially congested and later the wall becomes thickened, rubbery and haemorrhagic, while the lumen contains frank blood or sanguinous fluid. Arterial occlusion shows sharp demarcation (Fig. 51), while venous infarction is less well demarcated. Perforation may occur if untreated, but many patients may also die of shock. Incomplete occlusion less frequently results in infarction, but may cause patchy mucosal necrosis and superficial ulceration.

*Microscopical*   Early lesions (Fig. 52) are patchy and composed of mucosal necrosis overlain by mucus, fibrin, necrotic debris and blood cells. With increasing severity, ischaemic changes are seen in the deep layers of the bowel wall. Infarction (Fig. 53) is characterized by haemorrhage in the bowel wall, intravascular thrombosis and mucosal ulceration, sometimes with secondary infection. Healing at any stage may occur by resolution and formation of granulation tissue, often leading to fibrosis and stricture formation.

*Prognosis*   Depends upon duration of ischaemia, and whether surgical correction is possible or ischaemia reversible. Irreversible ischaemia will result in gangrene and /or perforation.

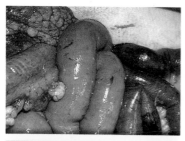

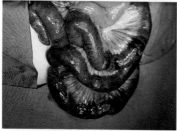

Fig. 50 Small intestine: acute infarction.

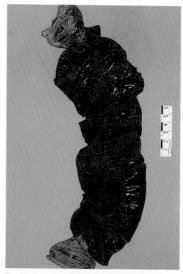

Fig. 51 Acute small bowel infarction due to arterial occlusion. Note sharp demarcation.

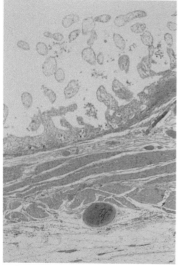

Fig. 52 Small intestine: acute ischaemia. H&E.

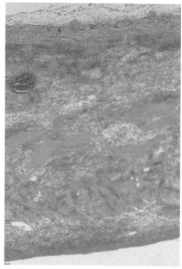

Fig. 53 Haemorrhagic infarction of bowel wall. H&E.

# 13 / **Bowel disorders of infancy**

## Hirschsprung's disease

*Incidence*  1 in 20 000–30 000 live births; M:F = 6–9:1.

*Aetiology*  Absence of ganglion cells in Meissner's and Auerbach's plexuses. Pre-existing non-myelinated nerve fibres undergo abnormal ramification.

*Macroscopical*  A narrow portion of aganglionic recto-sigmoid extending proximally from the anus, above which is an enormously dilated colon with a funnel shaped transition (Fig. 54).

*Microscopical*  Full-thickness rectal biopsy shows absent ganglion cells in plexuses of narrowed segment.

*Prognosis*  Unrelieved, causes proximal dilatation, possible rupture, enterocolitis and stercoral ulceration.

## Necrotizing enterocolitis

*Aetiology*  An ischaemic colitis in premature infants resulting from hypoxia, often with secondary bacterial infection.

*Macroscopical*  Patchy areas of haemorrhagic, friable, ulcerated mucosa with full-thickness necrosis (Fig. 55).

*Microscopical*  Necrosis, ulceration, haemorrhage and pneumatosis.

*Prognosis*  Depends on early treatment and infant's condition.

## Intussusception

*Aetiology*  In infancy there is usually no precipitating anatomical lesion, but an enlarged Peyer's patch due to a viral infection may form the apex.

*Macroscopical*  Telescoping of bowel into distal segment that may result in obstruction and strangulation (Figs 56 & 57).

*Prognosis*  Good if corrected before ischaemia intervenes.

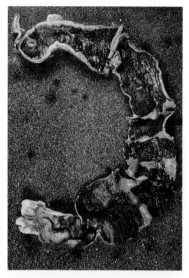

Fig. 54 Large intestine: Hirschsprung's disease.

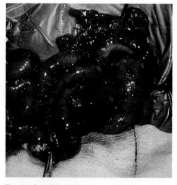

Fig. 55 Small intestine: necrotizing enterocolitis.

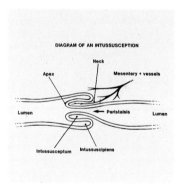

Fig. 56 Diagramatic representation of intussusception.

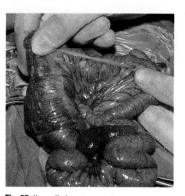

Fig. 57 Ileocolic intussusception.

# 14 / **Crohn's disease**

*Definition*  Chronic granulomatous disease, initially described as involving the terminal ileum (regional ileitis) but now known to affect any part of the bowel.

*Incidence*  Most commonly affects young adults, peak 20–30 yrs, but can appear at any age, even childhood or old age. M:F = 1:1. The incidence is increasing, especially in Northern Europe. It is rare in Africa and Asia.

*Aetiology*  Unknown. The histopathological picture suggests an inflammatory response to unidentified antigen such as a transmissable agent or gut contents.

*Macroscopical*  Distribution is often discontinuous, with 'skip lesions', consisting of areas of serpiginous aphthoid ulceration and marked oedema, thickening of bowel wall, often with stricture formation, serosal inflammation and fat wrapping. Fissuring of oedematous mucosa leaves isolated mucosal islands, producing the characteristic 'cobblestone' appearance (Fig. 58). Deep ulceration and fissuring can result in fistulation to neighbouring organs, e.g. other loops of bowel, bladder, skin, etc.

*Microscopical*  Involvement of full thickness of bowel wall. Oedema, ulceration and transmural inflammation, with focal collections of lymphocytes (Fig. 59). Occasional lymphoid follicles associated with fissuring and, in 50–70%, non-caseating epithelioid granulomas (Fig. 60) in the bowel wall and regional lymph nodes.

*Prognosis*  Recurrence after treatment is common and increases with length of follow-up. A progressive disorder with a high morbidity, often complicated by bowel obstruction, fistula formation, anaemia, ankylosing spondylitis, polyarthritis and liver disease. There is an increased incidence of carcinoma in affected small bowel.

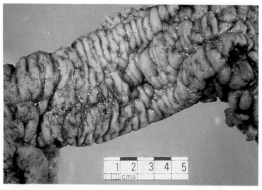

**Fig. 58** Thick bowel wall and cobblestone mucosa of Crohn's disease.

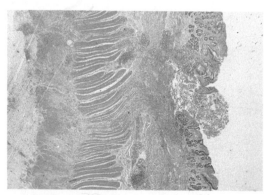

**Fig. 59** Crohn's disease. Note the transmural inflammation, ulceration and fissuring.

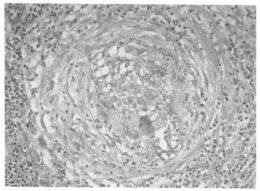

**Fig. 60** Non-caseating epithelioid granulomas associated with Crohn's disease.

# 15 / **Small bowel disorders**

## Coeliac disease (gluten-sensitive enteropathy)

*Aetiology*  A hypersensitivity reaction to gluten and its derivatives, causing malabsorption as a result of immunologically mediated mucosal damage. Hereditary influence is suggested by familial clustering and increased liability to form antireticulin antibodies.

*Macroscopical*  Loss of normal finger and/or leaf pattern of mucosa with villous atrophy characterized by a cribriform, mosaic or flat pattern.

*Microscopical*  Villi are severely blunted or distorted, with increased crypt depth and chronic inflammatory cell infiltrate in the lamina propria (Fig. 61). Similar changes may be seen in tropical sprue, cows' milk protein intolerance and disaccharidase deficiency.

*Prognosis*  Adherence to a gluten-free diet results in restoration of mucosal architecture and alleviation of symptoms. Complications may include small bowel lymphoma, carcinoma and dermatitis herpetiformis.

## Whipple's disease

Systemic disorder characterized by accumulation of macrophages showing cytoplasmic PAS-positive, diastase-resistant material. Electron microscopy shows minute intra- and extracellular bacilli.

*Incidence*  Usually Caucasians; M:F = 10:1. Most common in 4th or 5th decade.

*Macroscopical*  Thickened indurated small bowel wall with dulled serosa and prominent dilated lymphatics.

*Microscopical*  Lamina propria and villi are crowded and distorted by granular macrophages (Fig. 62).

*Prognosis*  Cured by antibiotics against presumed causative bacilli. Untreated it may be fatal.

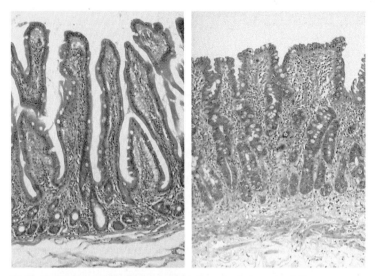

**Fig. 61** Jejunal biopsy: coeliac disease—subtotal villous atrophy (normal on left).

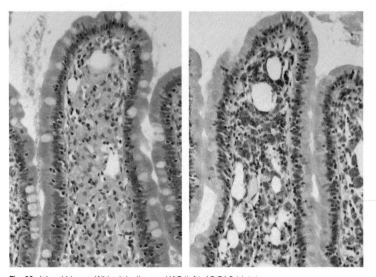

**Fig. 62** Jejunal biopsy: Whipple's disease. H&E (left), AB/PAS (right).

# 16 / **Diverticular disease**

*Definition*    Disorder typically affecting the sigmoid colon and characterized by acquired mucosal outpouchings associated with acquired abnormality of the intestinal muscle (Fig. 63).

*Incidence*    In Western society about 60% of those over 60 years of age have diverticular disease, with an increasing incidence with age. Uncommon in South America and rare in Africa, India and Asia.

*Aetiology*    Diverticula are most common in countries with a low roughage diet and are associated with marked thickening of portions of the circular muscle of the bowel wall. Evidence suggests abnormal contractility of large intestinal muscle with failure of relaxation, resulting in high intracolonic pressure zones and formation of pulsion diverticula at the sites where vessels pierce the muscularis propria.

*Macroscopical*    Two rows of diverticula are often identifiable between the mesenteric and antimesenteric taenia (Fig. 64); they consist of mucosa covered by muscularis mucosa and often containing faecoliths. There is associated thickening of the taenia and circular muscle (Fig. 65), giving a corrugated or concertina like appearance.

*Microscopical*    Diverticula lined by normal colonic mucosa, with an outer wall formed by muscularis mucosa lying between thickened bundles of circular muscularis propria broken up into fasciculi (Fig. 66). An acute inflammatory response is seen around the diverticula in diverticulitis.

*Prognosis*    Only about 20% of patients with diverticular disease suffer symptoms and of these only 20% suffer major complications such as inflammation (diverticulitis), perforation, haemorrhage (chronic from granulation tissue, or acute and massive from erosion of a submucosal vessel), fistula formation or intestinal obstruction.

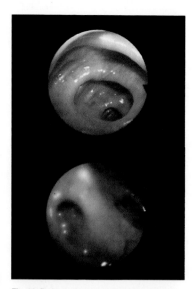

**Fig. 63** Endoscopic appearance of a colonic diverticulum.

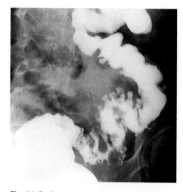

**Fig. 64** Radiological appearance of sigmoid diverticular disease on barium enema.

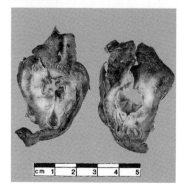

**Fig. 65** Diverticular disease: sigmoid colon in cross section, demonstrating diverticulum.

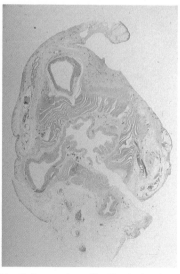

**Fig. 66** Same section as Fig. 65 stained to show relationship of diverticulum to muscularis.

# 17 / **Ulcerative colitis**

*Definition*     A recurrent inflammatory disorder of unknown aetiology affecting the large bowel.

*Incidence*     Worldwide distribution, but more common in USA, UK and Scandinavia where the incidence is 4–6/100 000. M:F = 2:3. Peak onset is in the 3rd decade, but the disorder may present in childhood or middle age.

*Aetiology*     Unknown, but 25% familial incidence and prevalence of HLA B27 in patients with ulcerative colitis and ankylosing spondylitis suggest a genetic influence. No organism has been isolated, but *E. coli* type 014 has surface antigens similar to alimentary glycoprotein, raising the possibility of cross reactivity. Cows' milk protein allergy has also been suggested.

*Macroscopical*     Mucosa is hyperaemic and oedematous, with numerous focal mucosal haemorrhages. The muscularis is spared, with no fissuring or fibrosis. In chronic cases, undermined mucosal margins and irregular, coalesced, broad-based ulcers result in pseudopolyp formation (Fig. 67).

*Microscopical*     Changes are limited to the mucosa: dense mixed inflammatory cell infiltrate, vascular congestion, depletion of goblet cells, glandular distortion and ulceration (Fig. 68). Crypt abscesses formed by polymorphs are a characteristic but non-specific feature (Fig. 69).

*Prognosis*     Most patients suffer a remitting, relapsing disorder marked by attacks of bloody diarrhoea. Some suffer a fulminant episode, which can be life threatening (toxic megacolon) (Fig. 70). There is a well recognized risk of colonic carcinoma in patients with longstanding (10 years) total chronic colitis. Patients at risk should be screened for premalignant dysplastic change.

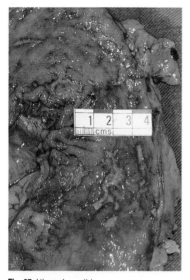

**Fig. 67** Ulcerative colitis.

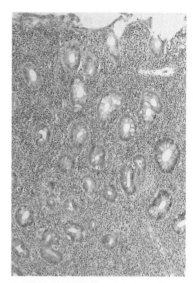

**Fig. 68** Ulcerative colitis: note inflammation limited to lamina propria.

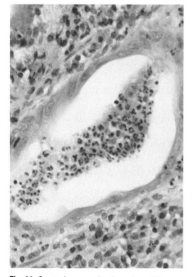

**Fig. 69** Crypt abscesses in ulcerative colitis.

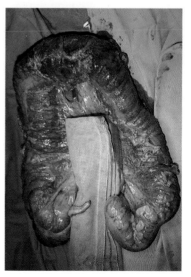

**Fig. 70** Ulcerative colitis: toxic megacolon.

# 18 / **Polyps of the colorectum**

*Introduction*    The majority are mucosal in origin, but hamartomatous Peutz–Jeghers and juvenile polyps also occur. Certain mesenchymal lesions, e.g. leiomyoma, haemangioma, lipoma and lymphoid lesions, may present as polyps.

## Metaplastic polyp

*Incidence*    Common incidental finding in rectosigmoid of adults in 6th or 7th decade. Often multiple.

*Aetiology*    Unknown. No proven relationship to malignancy.

*Macroscopical*    Smooth, round, sessile lesions, less than 5 mm.

*Microscopical*    Well formed glands and crypts of non-neoplastic mature goblet cells. Crowding of cells results in serrated luminal border. Foci of adenomatous change may be seen in large lesions.

*Significance*    Importance lies in differentiation from adenomas.

## Adenomatous polyps

*Incidence*    Found in 10% of necropsies and in 25% of patients with synchronous colorectal carcinoma.

*Macroscopical*    ***Tubular adenoma:*** pedunculated polyp with lobulated surface (Fig. 71).
***Villous adenoma:*** sessile papillary tumour with numerous fronds (Fig. 72).
***Tubulovillous:*** features of both.

*Microscopical*    ***Tubular adenoma:*** (Fig. 73) closely packed tubules with varying degree of dysplasia.
***Villous adenoma:*** (Fig. 74) fronds of fibrovascular tissue with dysplastic epithelium.
***Tubulovillous:*** intermediate features with short villous processes.

*Behaviour*    Malignant change is a risk in all adenomas, especially those >2 cm with a villous pattern. Malignant change found in 3–5% tubular adenomas, 15% of tubulovillous adenomas and 30–40% of villous adenomas.

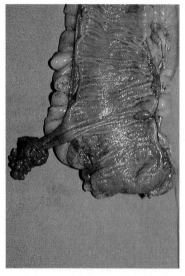

**Fig. 71** Typical pedunculated tubular adenoma.

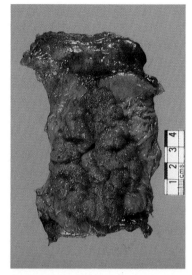

**Fig. 72** Typical sessile villous adenoma.

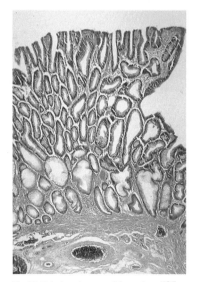

**Fig. 73** Tubular adenoma of the rectum. H&E.

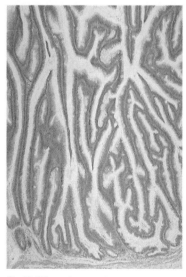

**Fig. 74** Villous adenoma of the rectum. H&E.

# 19 / **Tumours of the colorectum**

*Introduction*  Most colorectal tumours are epithelial in origin, but malignant counterparts of lipoma, leiomyoma and angioma can be seen. Along with lymphoma and carcinoid tumours, they account for 2% of large bowel tumours.

## Carcinoma

*Incidence*  Accounts for 18 000 deaths per annum in UK. Second to lung cancer in men and breast cancer in women as cause of death from cancer.

*Aetiology*  Many arise from pre-existing adenomatous polyps or in dysplastic areas as in ulcerative colitis.

*Macroscopical*  Ulcerated annular constricting lesions, or fungating polypoid masses (Fig. 75). About 70% of colonic cancers occur in rectosigmoid.

*Microscopical*  Well, moderate or poorly differentiated adenocarcinomas (Fig. 76) with variable amounts of extracellular mucin. Mucinous carcinomas (Fig. 77), undifferentiated and signet ring variants are also recognized. Squamous carcinoma is limited to the anal canal.

*Prognosis*  Extent of spread and presence of node metastases, as reflected in Duke's staging, provide the best prognostic index. Degree of differentiation and presence of local vascular invasion are also a guide.

## Familial polyposis coli

This is an autosomal dominant inherited condition characterized by multiple adenomatous polyps (Fig. 78) in late teenage or early adult life. Malignant change is inevitable in untreated cases and therefore total colectomy in teenage is necessary. Similar polyps may also be found in the stomach, duodenum and small bowel.

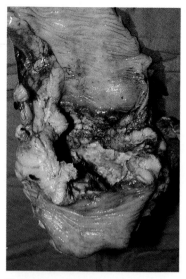

**Fig. 75** Ulcerated fungating carcinoma of the colon.

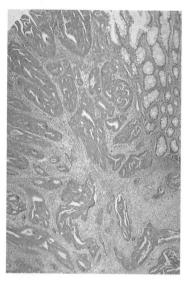

**Fig. 76** Adenocarcinoma of the colon.

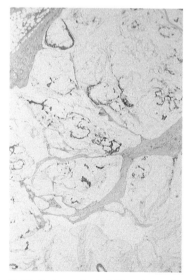

**Fig. 77** Mucin secreting (colloid) carcinoma of the colon. H&E.

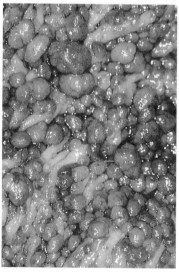

**Fig. 78** Familial polyposis coli: mucosa studded with multiple adenomatous polyps.

# 20 / **Miscellaneous disorders of the colorectum**

## Melanosis coli

*Definition*     Characterized by melanin-like pigmentation of the colonic mucosa.

*Incidence*     Previously about 10% of necropsies, but now falling with declining use of anthracene purgatives.

*Aetiology*     Related to chronic constipation and anthracene purgative consumption. Current evidence suggests pigment is lipofuscin from damaged cellular organelles.

*Macroscopical*     The colonic mucosa is coloured from black to varying shades of brown (Fig. 79). The right colon is more affected than the left, but the ileum is never involved.

*Microscopical*     The lamina propria contains numerous macrophages laden with golden-brown pigment. In severe cases, macrophages extend into the submucosa (Fig. 80).

## Solitary rectal ulcer

*Definition*     Characterized by anterior or anterolateral, flat and well-demarcated irregular ulcers (despite the name) occasionally covered by white slough. Sometimes there is no ulcer but proctitis with mucosal roughening and irregularity.

*Aetiology*     Possibly from mucosal prolapse, trauma or ischaemia from excessive straining.

*Microscopical*     Obliteration of lamina propria by fibrosis and upward growth of smooth muscle fibres from a thickened muscularis mucosa. Superficial ulceration with crypt irregularity, epithelial hyperplasia and goblet cell depletion (Fig. 81).

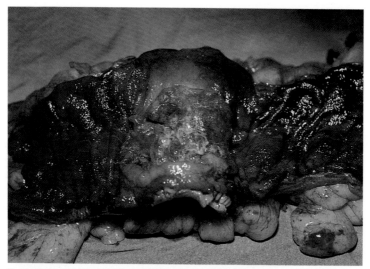

**Fig. 79** Melanosis coli with carcinoma. Note uniform black pigmentation of colonic mucosa.

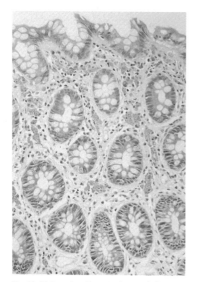

**Fig. 80** Melanosis coli: note pigment-laden macrophages in lamina propria. H&E ×64.

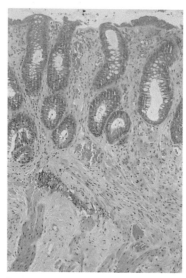

**Fig. 81** Solitary rectal ulcer. Note fraying and splaying of muscularis mucosa. H&E ×64.

# 21 / **The appendix**

## Acute appendicitis

*Incidence*    Extremely common, occurring from infancy to old age, with peak incidence in 2nd and 3rd decades.

*Aetiology*    Common in Western society. Usually resulting from luminal obstruction by a faecolith, lymphoid hypertrophy or foreign material.

*Macroscopical*    Tense, turgid, distended erythematous appendix (Fig. 82) covered with purulent exudate. If neglected, necrosis occurs with perforation.

*Microscopical*    Polymorphonuclear infiltration with epithelial ulceration, oedema of the wall and later coagulative necrosis (Fig. 83).

*Prognosis*    Excellent after early appendicectomy (mortality <0.1%). Delay in treatment is associated with increased morbidity (peritonitis, pelvic or subphrenic abscess, septicaemia). Occasionally, spontaneous resolution can lead to progressive fibrosis and luminal obliteration (Fig. 84).

## Carcinoid of the appendix

*Incidence*    Found in 0.1% of all appendices examined, representing 85% of all appendiceal tumours.

*Aetiology*    Unknown. Arises from enterochromaffin cells.

*Macroscopical*    Firm yellow tumour often with superimposed acute inflammation.

*Microscopical*    Nests of uniform cells with well-defined periphery and a fibrous stroma (Fig. 85).

*Spread*    Rare apart from para-appendiceal nodes. Distant metastases occur in <0.1% and are related to size of tumour.

*Prognosis*    Good following excision.

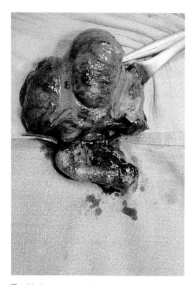

**Fig. 82** Acute appendicitis.

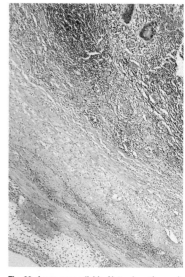

**Fig. 83** Acute appendicitis. Note ulceration and transmural acute inflammation. H&E ×25.

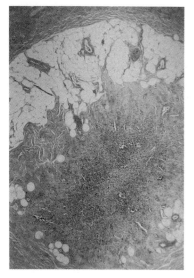

**Fig. 84** Appendiceal fibrosis with luminal obliteration due to previous inflammation. H&E.

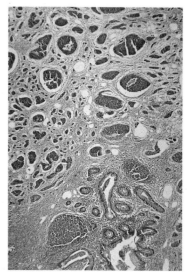

**Fig. 85** Appendix: carcinoid tumour.

# 22 / **Hepatitis**

Hepatitis may be due to infectious agents, including viruses type A, type B and non-A non-B, or toxins, including alcohol, carbon tetrachloride, halothane and paracetamol.

## Acute hepatitis

*Macroscopical* — Dusky red enlargement in lobular hepatitis or later red patchy areas with softening and brown/green discoloration of massive necrosis.

*Microscopical* — Diffuse portal tract inflammation with lymphocytes and histiocytes, extending into lobules, with foci of liver cell necrosis and Kupffer cell hyperplasia (Fig. 86). Confluent areas of necrosis between hepatic veins and portal triads may be seen, with massive necrosis in fulminant cases such as those due to paracetamol poisoning.

## Chronic hepatitis

*Definition* — Persistent hepatic inflammation for over 6 months.

*Aetiology* — Viral, drug-induced, idiopathic.

### Chronic persistent hepatitis

*Microscopical* — Mononuclear inflammatory cell infiltrate of portal tracts (Fig. 87), with normal architecture and intact border between portal tract and lobules (limiting plate), with only minimal fibrosis and cell necrosis. It may follow acute viral hepatitis; progression to cirrhosis is not seen, but chronic active hepatitis may develop.

### Chronic active hepatitis

*Microscopical* — Marked portal tract inflammation destroying limiting plate with necrosis, degeneration and regeneration of hepatocytes and early fibrosis, often progressing to cirrhosis. In some cases it may follow viral hepatitis (B and non-A non-B), but some have serological abnormalities (lupoid hepatitis) suggesting an autoimmune aetiology.

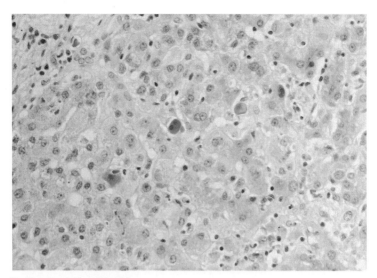

**Fig. 86** Acute viral hepatitis. H&E.

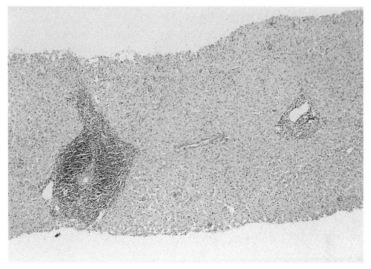

**Fig. 87** Chronic persistent hepatitis. H&E.

# 23 / **Alcoholic liver disease**

Excess alcohol consumption can result in fatty liver (steatosis), alcoholic hepatitis, cirrhosis and liver cell carcinoma.

*Incidence*    Fatty liver is almost invariable, but is non-specific and reversible. Hepatitis occurs in about 33% of alcoholics, but can subside or progress to cirrhosis. Cirrhosis occurs in 10–15% of alcoholics and is progressive. About 15% of cirrhotics develop carcinoma.

*Aetiology*    The exact mechanism of alcoholic damage is poorly understood. It is hepatotoxic, deranging lipogenesis, NADH:NAD ratio and cholesterol metabolism, thus resulting in steatosis. The mechanisms of hepatitis and fibrogenesis producing cirrhosis are unknown.

*Macroscopical*    ***Fatty liver*** is enlarged, pale and greasy to touch with obscured lobular markings.

***Alcoholic hepatitis:*** non-specific hepatomegaly.

***Alcoholic cirrhosis*** is usually micronodular but may be macronodular in the late stages.

*Microscopical*    ***Fatty liver:*** (Fig. 88) intracellular accumulation of lipid in hepatocytes, producing large cytoplasmic vacuoles with displacement of the nucleus. Adjacent cell membranes may rupture to form fat cysts, and the rupture of these results in lipogranuloma formation.

***Alcoholic hepatitis:*** (Fig. 89) focal hepatocyte necrosis associated with a neutrophil polymorph reaction. There is steatosis, often with lipogranulomata, Kupffer cell hyperplasia and a light chronic inflammatory cell infiltrate. Mallory's hyaline (Fig. 90) (intracytoplasmic aggregates of glassy red material) is frequently seen. Fibrosis around central veins extending into lobules is often present.

***Alcoholic cirrhosis:*** the features are the same as any cirrhosis, but with aetiological clues such as Mallory's hyaline formation.

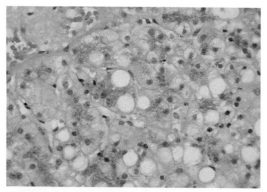

**Fig. 88** Liver: fatty change. Numerous intracytoplasmic fat droplets. H&E.

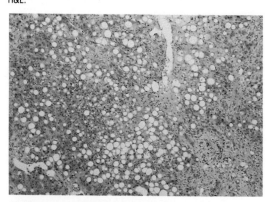

**Fig. 89** Liver: acute alcoholic hepatitis. H&E.

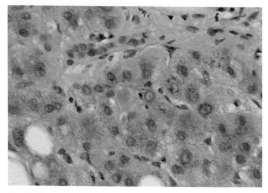

**Fig. 90** Liver: acute alcoholic hepatitis—Mallory's hyaline formation. H&E.

# 24 / **Hepatic cirrhosis**

*Definition*    An irreversible condition of the liver in which the normal lobular architecture is destroyed and replaced by numerous nodules showing focal necrosis and regeneration separated by fibrois tissue septae.

*Aetiology*
- Cryptogenic (40%).
- Alcoholic (30%).
- Post-hepatitic (including chronic active hepatitis progressing to cirrhosis—15%).
- Biliary cirrhosis.
- Metabolic and inherited conditions, e.g. haemachromatosis, Wilson's disease, thalassaemia, $\alpha_1$-antitrypsin deficiency, galactosaemia, type IV glycogen storage disease, tyrosinosis, fructose intolerance (5%).
- Drugs, e.g. methotrexate.
- Venous outflow obstruction, i.e. Budd-Chiari syndrome.

*Macroscopical*
- Micronodular (Fig. 91) nodules of similar size, usually <3 mm diameter.
- Macronodular (Fig. 92) nodules varying in size, but usually >3 mm and <1 cm.
- Mixed: features of both forms of cirrhosis.

*Microscopical*    Nodules of liver tissue separated by fibrous septae (Fig. 93), with variable bile duct proliferation and inflammation. Vascular architecture is distorted and destroyed and there is evidence of hepatocyte necrosis and regeneration. Mallory's hyaline or bile duct granulomata may suggest the underlying aetiology.

*Prognosis*    Established cirrhosis is irreversible. Complications include hepatocellular failure, portal hypertension and hepatocellular carcinoma.

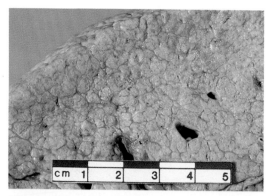

**Fig. 91** Micronodular hepatic cirrhosis.

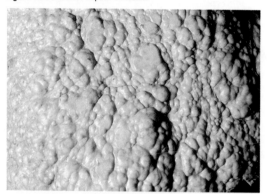

**Fig. 92** Macronodular hepatic cirrhosis.

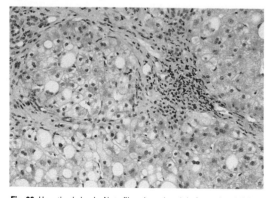

**Fig. 93** Hepatic cirrhosis. Note fibrosis and nodule formation. H&E.

# 25 / **Biliary cirrhosis**

Biliary cirrhosis results from prolonged cholestasis of intra- or extrahepatic origin.

## Primary biliary cirrhosis

*Aetiology*    Probably an autoimmune disorder resulting in non-suppurative inflammatory destruction of septal and interlobar bile ducts. It occurs in middle-aged women in association with other autoimmune disorders, and abnormalities of humoral and cell-mediated immunity (typically a high titre of antimitochondrial antibodies).

*Macroscopical*    Liver is slightly enlarged, deeply bile pigmented with regular micronodular scarring.

*Microscopical*    Cholangioles and interlobar bile ducts show epithelial degeneration, tangling, knotting and luminal obliteration, associated with dense mononuclear cell inflammation and sarcoid-like granuloma in about half the cases (Fig. 94). Inflammation may extend around periportal hepatocytes, where there is usually evidence of cholesterosis. Mallory's hyaline is found in 25%.

*Prognosis*    Depends on degree of scarring. The disease usually has a slowly progressive course, ending in liver failure.

## Secondary biliary cirrhosis

*Aetiology*    Results from obstruction to extrahepatic ducts.

*Microscopical*    Bile accumulation in hepatocytes, canaliculi and Kuppfer cells and dilatation of bile ducts filled with inspissated bile. Later, bile duct proliferation (Fig. 95) and chronic portal tract inflammation are seen, with necrotic pigment-laden cells (bile infarcts) and bile leakage from ruptured canals of Hering (bile lakes). Ascending cholangitis may be superimposed.

*Prognosis*    Hepatic failure is the usual outcome.

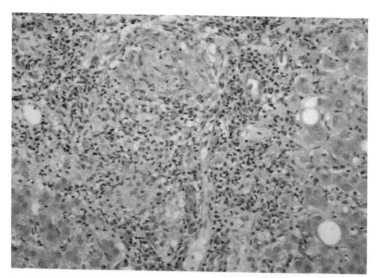

**Fig. 94** Primary biliary cirrhosis. H&E. Note granuloma formation with destruction of ducts.

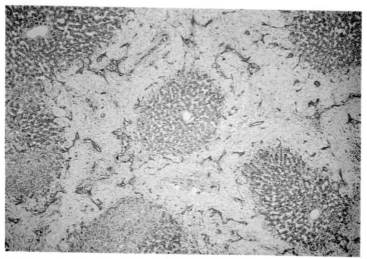

**Fig. 95** Secondary biliary cirrhosis: fibrosis and ductule proliferation in portal tracts. H&E.

# 26 / **Benign tumours of the liver**

Benign tumours may arise from any of the cellular constituents of the liver, but the most frequent are liver cell adenoma (LCA) and focal nodular hyperplasia (FNH).

*Incidence*  Both LCA and FNH have increased in incidence in recent years, but still remain uncommon. LCA usually occurs in women of childbearing age.

*Aetiology*  Development of LCA and FNH has been associated with gonadal steroid therapy and, in particular, the contraceptive pill. Risk of developing LCA in a woman on the pill is related to age, years of use and the dose of both oestrogen and progesterone components.

## Liver cell adenoma

*Macroscopical*  Usually single, well defined, yellowish nodules 2–15 cm in diameter in otherwise normal livers. Rupture with intraperitoneal haemorrhage occurs in about 25%.

*Microscopical*  Consists of hepatocytes in closely packed trabeculae 2 or 3 cells thick, separated by narrow sinusoids. Tumour cells are large, with small uniform nuclei and clear cytoplasm containing excess fat or glycogen. Fibrous tracts and bile ducts are absent (Fig. 96).

*Prognosis*  Rupture and intraperitoneal haemorrhage may be fatal; local excision is curative.

## Focal nodular hyperplasia

*Macroscopical*  A solitary globular mass, up to about 5 cm, bulging beneath the liver surface (Fig. 97). Rupture is uncommon.

*Microscopical*  Nodules of hepatocytes separated by fibrous trabeculae containing bile ducts and small vessels radiating from a central stellate fibrous scar (Fig. 98). Multiple FNH, occupying much of the liver in the perihilar region, is called partial nodular transformation.

*Prognosis*  Local excision is curative.

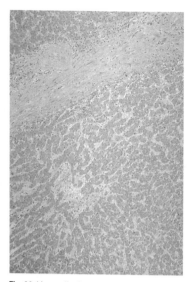

**Fig. 96** Liver cell adenoma.

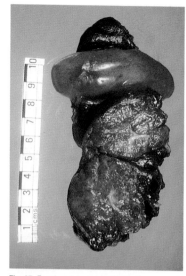

**Fig. 97** Focal nodular hyperplasia. Note central stellate scar.

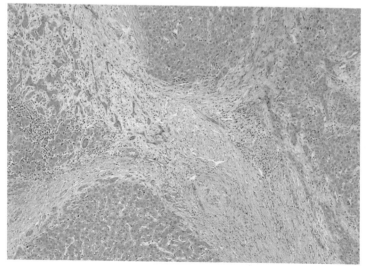

**Fig. 98** Focal nodular hyperplasia. H&E ×10.

# 27 / Malignant tumours of the liver

## Primary tumours

Of primary tumours, hepatocellular carcinoma accounts for 85%, cholangiocarcinoma 10% and the rest 5%.

### Hepatocellular carcinoma

*Aetiology*    In the UK this usually occurs in established cirrhosis, and especially in cirrhosis associated with hepatitis B infection.

*Macroscopical*    Single large mass of partly necrotic, haemorrhagic, bile-stained tissue (Fig. 99). Can be multifocal; vascular invasion is common.

*Microscopical*    Malignant hepatocytes of varying differentiation arranged in trabecular, pseudoglandular or scirrhous pattern (Fig. 100).

*Prognosis*    Few survivals after excision; the condition is usually fatal.

### Haemangiosarcoma

*Aetiology*    Rare. It occurs in those exposed to the contrast medium Thorotrast, vinyl chloride monomer or arsenic.

*Macroscopical*    Multiple, ill-defined masses throughout liver.

*Microscopical*    Blood-filled channels formed by malignant endothelial cells (Fig. 101).

*Prognosis*    Widespread blood-borne metastases. Survival is rare.

## Secondary tumours

Most liver neoplasms are secondary. Liver is a common site for metastatic carcinoma, melanoma, sarcoma, leukaemia and lymphoma.

*Macroscopical*    Either multiple umbilicated masses (carcinoma, melanoma, sarcoma) (Fig. 102) or diffuse infiltration (leukaemia, lymphoma).

*Microscopical*    Deposits and infiltrates resembling primary.

*Prognosis*    Most die within 1 yr.

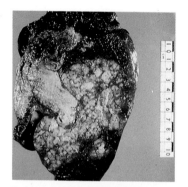

Fig. 99 Hepatocellular carcinoma.

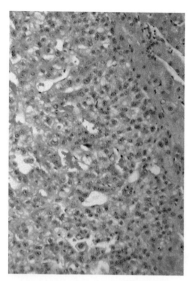

Fig. 100 Hepatocellular carcinoma. Note cords and sheets of atypical hepatocytes. H&E.

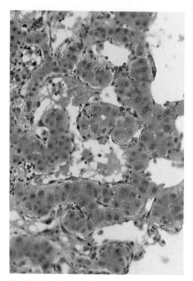

Fig. 101 Liver haemangiosarcoma. Vascular spaces lined by neoplastic endothelial cells. H&E ×25.

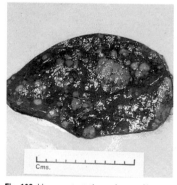

Fig. 102 Liver: metastatic carcinoma. Note umbilication of subcapsular tumour deposits.

# 28 / Tumours of bile ducts and gallbladder

Benign epithelial tumours, e.g. papilloma or adenoma, are rare and result from localized epithelial overgrowth. They are usually incidental findings but may produce obstructive symptoms. Mesenchymal tumours also occur but are very rare.

## Cholangiocarcinoma

*Incidence*    1% of all carcinomas. M:F = 1:4. Peak age of incidence: 60–70 yrs.

*Aetiology*    Increased incidence in chronic inflammatory bowel disease, congenital duct abnormalities, e.g. choledochal cyst, *Clonorchis sinensis* infection.

*Macroscopical*    Occurs anywhere from intrahepatic bile ducts down to ampulla of Vater. Intrahepatic tumours present in similar manner to hepatocellular carcinoma; extrahepatic tumours produce obstructive jaundice. Scirrhous growths spread along ducts and produce strictures (Fig. 103).

*Microscopical*    Well or moderately differentiated adenocarcinoma in abundant fibrous stroma with perineural infiltration. It may be difficult to distinguish from metastatic tumour without in situ change in adjacent ducts (Fig. 104).

*Prognosis*    Slowly progressive, but ultimately poor outcome.

## Carcinoma of the gallbladder

*Aetiology*    Cholelithiasis and cholecystitis are present in 75–90%. Cholic acid derivatives are powerful experimental carcinogens.

*Macroscopical*    Infiltrating mass, often involving liver.

*Microscopical*    About 90% adenocarcinoma (Fig. 105), with a few adenosquamous or squamous carcinomas arising in metaplastic epithelium.

*Prognosis*    Often symptomless until spread to liver or ducts. Resection seldom possible. 5% survival at 5 yrs.

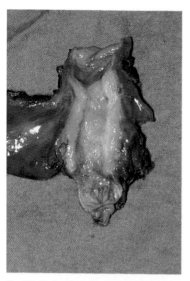

**Fig. 103** Cholangiocarcinoma. Malignant stricture in common bile duct.

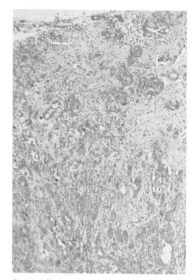

**Fig. 104** Cholangiocarcinoma. H & E.

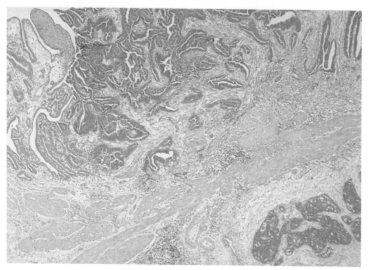

**Fig. 105** Primary adenocarcinoma of the gallbladder.

# 29 / Cholelithiasis

| | |
|---|---|
| *Incidence* | Frequent in Western Caucasians, especially obese middle-aged women. |
| *Aetiology* | Mechanism unknown. The predisposing causes include:<br>• changes in bile composition<br>• local factors in gallbladder<br>• biliary tract infection. |
| *Macroscopical* | • Mixed stones of cholesterol, bile pigment, calcium salts and organic material (Fig. 106)<br>• Pure cholesterol stones<br>• Bile pigment stones associated with haemolysis. |
| *Presentation* | May be silent or present as biliary colic, cholecystitis, obstructive jaundice, gallstone ileus, pancreatitis and gallbladder carcinoma. |

## Acute cholecystitis

Acute inflammation initiated by stone impaction with hyperconcentration of bile and an initial chemical inflammation and secondary infection.

| | |
|---|---|
| *Macroscopical* | Enlarged, tense, red or violaceous gallbladder with serosal fibrinopurulent exudate. |
| *Microscopical* | Mucosal ulceration, transmural acute inflammation and cellular exudate of neutrophils with fibrinous exudate, oedema and congestion (Fig. 107). |
| *Course* | Resolution, progression to chronic cholecystitis or complications such as empyema or gangrenous necrosis. |

## Chronic cholecystitis

| | |
|---|---|
| *Macroscopical* | Thickened contracted gallbladder with stones. |
| *Microscopical* | Mucosal ulceration, reactive proliferation and foci of metaplasia. Mononuclear inflammatory infiltrate, fibrous thickening and prominent intramural herniations of epithelium (Fig. 108) are also present (Rokitansky-Aschoff sinuses). Complex overgrowth of multiple sinuses known as adenomyomatosis. |

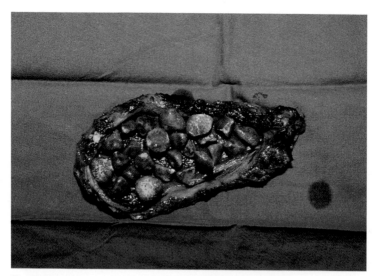

**Fig. 106** Gallstones.

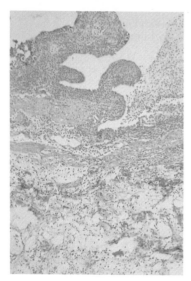

**Fig. 107** Gallbladder: acute cholecystitis. H&E.

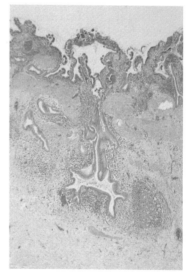

**Fig. 108** Gallbladder: chronic cholecystitis with Rokitansky-Aschoff sinuses. H&E.

# 30 / **Pancreatitis**

## Acute pancreatitis

Diffuse destruction of pancreatic tissue by escape of activated pancreatic enzymes.

*Incidence*     More common over age of 40. M:F = 1:3 in Britain.

*Aetiology*     Biliary disease (50%) and excess alcohol (20%) are the most important predisposing factors. Others include trauma, mumps, hypothermia, ischaemia, hyperparathyroidism, hyperlipidaemia and drugs (thiazides, sulphonamides, azathioprine).

*Macroscopical*     Areas of grey proteolytic necrosis, haemorrhage, and white foci of fat necrosis seen in adjacent mesentery or omentum (Fig. 109). There is often a blood-stained serous peritoneal exudate.

*Microscopical*     Granular coagulative necrosis of pancreatic tissue, inflammatory cell exudate, fibrinoid necrosis of vessels and haemorrhage (Fig. 110), with local fat necrosis.

*Outcome*     Often circulatory collapse with high mortality. It may lead to abscess or pseudocyst formation.

## Chronic pancreatitis

*Incidence*     More common in males.

*Aetiology*     Similar for acute pancreatitis, but excess alcohol intake is more frequently implicated.

*Macroscopical*     Pancreas is usually hard and shrunken, but may be enlarged. Often visible foci of calcification.

*Microscopical*     Destructive inter- and intralobular fibrosis, mononuclear cell infiltrate, and epithelial atrophy, with duct dilatation, foci of squamous metaplasia and calculi formation. Islets of Langerhans are often well preserved (Fig. 111).

*Outcome*     Pain, duct obstruction, pancreatic insufficiency, malabsorption and, often, diabetes mellitus.

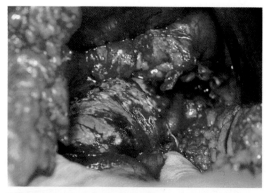

**Fig. 109** Acute haemorrhagic pancreatitis. Operative photograph.

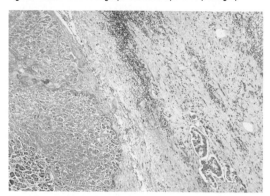

**Fig. 110** Acute pancreatitis. Note lobular necrosis, haemorrhage and inflammation. H&E.

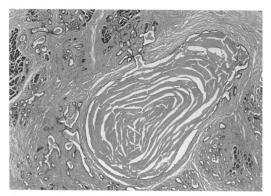

**Fig. 111** Chronic pancreatitis. Note lobular atrophy, fibrosis and chronic inflammation. H&E.

# 31 / **Tumours of the pancreas**

Although benign tumours (e.g. cystadenoma) are seen, the majority are carcinomas arising from the exocrine pancreas, with a few islet cell tumours of variable behaviour.

## Carcinoma of the pancreas

*Incidence*  Threefold increase in last 40 yrs in UK, with 5700 deaths/yr. M:F = 2:1, 90% occur from 6th decade onwards.

*Aetiology*  Smoking increases risk by 2.5 times. Excess dietary fat, coffee consumption and exposure to certain chemicals have also been implicated.

*Macroscopical*  Majority occur in the head, the rest in the body or tail, or diffusely infiltrate the entire organ. Grey scirrhous tumour (Fig. 112) which may invade duodenum, bile duct and adjacent tissues.

*Microscopical*  Adenocarcinomas of varying differentiation and mucin secretion (Fig. 113), typically set in a dense fibrous stroma. Acinar, anaplastic and cystic (cyst-adenocarcinoma) variants are seen. Perineural lymphatic invasion is common.

*Prognosis*  Poor, most dying within 6 mths. May produce obstructive jaundice and invade local organs. Nodal and hepatic metastases are frequent.

## Islet cell tumours

Occur mainly in adults, may be single or multiple, hormonally active or non-functional, benign or malignant. They may also be associated with the multiple endocrine adenoma (MEA) syndrome.

*Macroscopical*  Yellow/brown nodules varying greatly in size.

*Microscopical*  Cords and nests of well differentiated islet cells, with electron dense granules. Difficult to predict behaviour from histology (Fig. 114).

*Function*  Can produce insulin, gastrin (Zollinger-Ellison syndrome), glucagon, VIP and somatostatin.

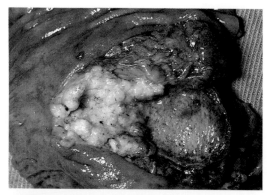

**Fig. 112** Adenocarcinoma of the pancreas.

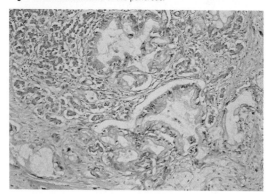

**Fig. 113** Pancreas: primary ductal adenocarcinoma. H&E.

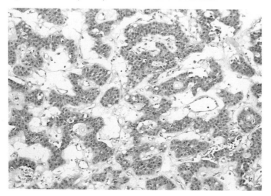

**Fig. 114** Pancreas islet cell tumour. H&E.

# 32 / Kidney: hydronephrosis and vesicoureteric reflux

## Hydronephrosis

*Definition*   Dilatation of renal pelvis and calyces.

*Aetiology*   Bilateral hydronephrosis follows urethral or bilateral ureteric obstruction or neurogenic disturbance of bladder control. Unilateral cases follow congenital pelviureteric obstruction or ureteric obstruction (e.g. stones or tumour).

*Macroscopical*   Gradual onset causes pelvicalyceal distension, with irregular atrophy of renal substance, and fibrosis with a lobulated surface (Fig. 115).

*Microscopical*   Longstanding cases result in tubular atrophy, interstitial fibrosis and glomerular atrophy. Superimposed pyelonephritis may be present.

*Prognosis*   Depends on the underlying obstructing pathology and the speed of relief. Unrelieved cases may die in renal failure.

## Vesicoureteric reflux

*Definition*   Retrograde propulsion of urine up the ureter during micturition. It is seen in 30–50% of children with recurrent urinary infections.

*Aetiology*   Congenital abnormality of oblique entry of ureter into bladder; may be associated with urethral valves, megacystis and megaureter, duplex ureters and ureteric ectopia.

*Macroscopical*   There is calyceal dilatation (clubbing) and wedge shaped parenchymal scars (Fig. 116). Refluxing papillae are characterized by a concave surface and round, rather than slit-like, duct openings.

*Microscopical*   Widespread tubular atrophy, interstitial fibrosis, chronic inflammatory infiltrate and lymphoid follicles.

*Prognosis*   Renal failure in late childhood if untreated.

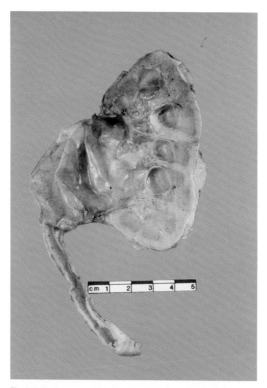

**Fig. 115** Hydronephrosis. The lower end of the ureter is obstructed by tumour.

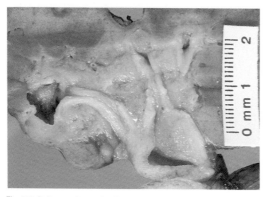

**Fig. 116** Reflux nephropathy. Scarring tends to be located at poles of kidney. H&E.

## Acute pyelonephritis

*Definition*    Acute bacterial infection of the kidney.

*Incidence*    Common in infancy, childhood, pregnancy and old age. It is more common in women.

*Aetiology*    Ascending infection of urinary tract, often predisposed to by urinary tract abnormalities (e.g. reflux, obstruction) and diabetes mellitus.

*Macroscopical*    Swollen hyperaemic kidney, with scattered round or linear abscesses extending from papillae to cortex with surface abscess formation (Fig. 117).

*Microscopical*    Extensive focal suppurative tubular destruction (Fig. 118) with polymorphs in adjacent tubules but glomerular sparing.

*Complications*    Renal failure, perinephric abscess, carbuncle, papillary necrosis, pyonephrosis and chronic pyelonephritis.

## Chronic pyelonephritis

*Definition*    Chronic inflammation of renal parenchyma from persisting infection.

*Macroscopical*    Small irregular scarred kidneys with discrete corticomedullary scars overlying dilated calyces with thick granular walls or atrophic mucosa (Fig. 119). Scarring is most marked at poles when associated with vesicoureteric reflux.

*Microscopical*    Tubular atrophy interspersed with dilated tubules filled with colloid eosinophilic casts (thyroidization) plus interstitial inflammation, periglomerular fibrosis, obliterative endarteritis and ischaemic scarring (Fig. 120).

*Complications*    Hypertension, chronic renal failure.

## Renal tuberculosis

Blood-borne spread manifesting as miliary, fibrocaseous or tuberculous pyonephrosis.

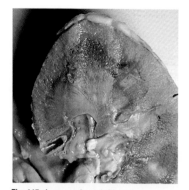

**Fig. 117** Acute pyelonephritis.

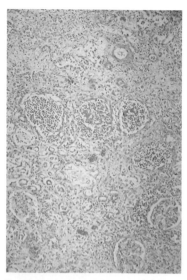

**Fig. 118** Acute pyelonephritis. Note intratubular collections of polymorphs. H&E.

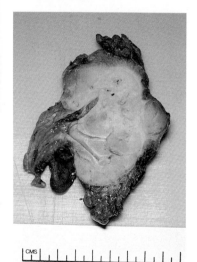

**Fig. 119** Chronic pyelonephritis. Note scarring and destruction of pyramids.

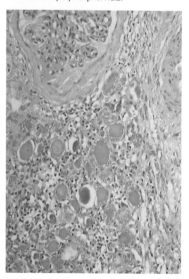

**Fig. 120** Chronic pyelonephritis. Typical 'thyroidization' of renal tubules. H&E.

# 34 / **Urinary calculi**

Urinary calculi form by precipitation of urinary constituents associated with small fragments of organic material.

*Stone types*   Three types of calculi are recognized:
- mixed uric acid and urate stones (form in acidic urine)
- calcium oxalate stones (form in acidic urine)
- complex triple phosphate stones composed of magnesium, ammonium and calcium carbonates (form in alkaline urine).

Calcium oxalate stones are the commonest.

*Aetiology*   Precipitation is favoured by highly concentrated urine and excess secretion of stone constituents.

*Macroscopical*   Urate stones are rounded, hard, brown and rarely larger than a few millimetres. Oxalate stones are irregular, hard and dark brown due to blood pigment. Triple phosphate stones are irregular, friable and whitish, and can attain a considerable size (Figs 121 & 122). All primary stones may also have secondary surface deposits resulting in compound or laminated stones.

*Sites*   Urinary calculi may form in the renal pelvis or bladder and may be single or multiple.

*Effects*   Stones can lead to mechanical effects causing pain (ureteric colic), intermittent obstruction (Fig. 123), irritation of the mucosa with haematuria, or mucosal ulceration and squamous metaplasia (which may carry the risk of development of squamous carcinoma). Stones are commonly associated with secondary infection.

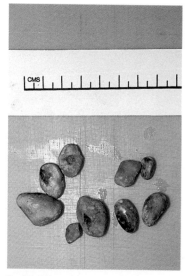

Fig. 121 Renal calculi.

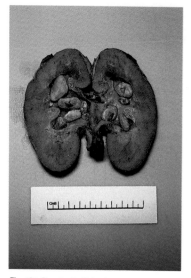

Fig. 122 Renal calculi, in situ.

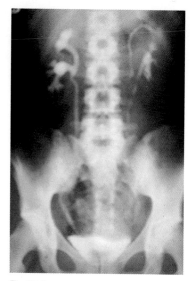

Fig. 123 Intravenous urogram. Stone obstructing right ureter. Duplex left ureter.

# 35 / Tumours of the kidneys

Benign tumours (e.g. cortical adenomas, fibromas) are usually insignificant, while angiomyolipomas and oncocytomas present as a renal mass, and juxtaglomerular cell tumours cause hypertension.

## Renal cell carcinoma (hypernephroma)

*Incidence*  1–3% of visceral malignancies and 85% of adult renal tumours. About 1500 deaths/yr.

*Macroscopical*  Lobulated, creamy yellow, variegated tumour with areas of necrosis and haemorrhage (Fig. 124).

*Microscopical*  Clear cells due to cytoplasmic lipid and glycogen content (Fig. 125), in papillary, solid or tubular form set in a delicate vascular stroma.

*Prognosis*  About 45% 5 yr survival. It depends on tumour size, venous and capsular invasion and degree of nuclear pleomorphism.

## Nephroblastoma (Wilms' tumour)

*Incidence*  Common visceral tumour in childhood (1–4 yrs).

*Macroscopical*  Mixture of soft, pale grey, fleshy tissue and cartilaginous tissue, with areas of haemorrhagic necrosis (Fig. 126).

*Microscopical*  Primitive glomeruli and abortive tubules in spindle cell stroma which may differentiate into muscle, bone, fat or cartilage (Fig. 127).

*Prognosis*  Combination treatment with surgery, chemo- and radiotherapy results in up to 90% 5 yr survival, depending on age, tumour stage and degree of differentiation.

## Transitional cell carcinoma (TCC) of renal pelvis

Similar aetiology to TCC in bladder and often associated with tumours elsewhere in the urinary tract.

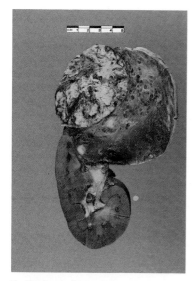

**Fig. 124** Renal adenocarcinoma.

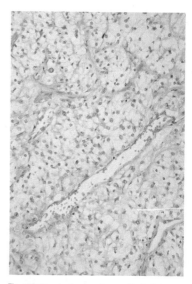

**Fig. 125** Renal adenocarcinoma. Typical clear cells. H&E.

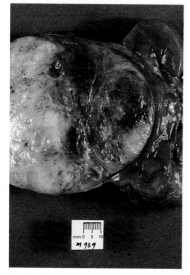

**Fig. 126** Nephroblastoma.

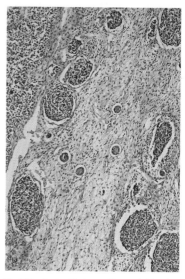

**Fig. 127** Nephroblastoma. Glomeruloid and tubular structures in mesenchymal stroma. H&E.

# 36 / Congenital abnormalities and inflammation of the urinary tract

## Congenital abnormalities

Double (duplex) ureters are occasional incidental findings. Exstrophy of the bladder (ectopia vesicae, Fig. 128), due to developmental failure of the anterior abdominal wall, is associated with ascending pyelonephritis, and development of adenocarcinoma.

## Inflammation

Acute and chronic cystitis and urethritis associated with urinary tract infection present no specific histological features. Cystitis may be catarrhal, purulent, pseudomembranous or granulomatous, e.g. tuberculosis, schistosomiasis.

## Malakoplakia

*Macroscopical*   Pale yellow mucosal plaques tending to ulcerate.

*Microscopical*   Granulation tissue containing macrophages with PAS-positive concentric cytoplasmic granules (Michaelis-Gutmann bodies) (Fig. 129) probably representing degenerate bacterial debris.

## Interstitial cystitis (Hunner's ulcer)

*Incidence*   A disease of adult females.

*Macroscopical*   Trigone oedema and ulceration with fissuring and haemorrhage during bladder distension.

*Microscopical*   Mucosal ulceration, fibrinous exudate, oedema and congestion of submucosa and muscularis with non-specific inflammatory infiltrate containing mast cells (Fig. 130).

## Schistosomiasis

Infection with *Schistosoma haematobium* results in a chronic granulomatous cystitis (Fig. 131). The mucosa often shows squamous metaplasia, and squamous carcinoma is an important complication in endemic areas of chronic schistosomiasis.

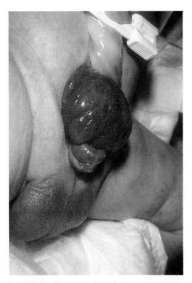

**Fig. 128** Bladder: ectopia vesicae.

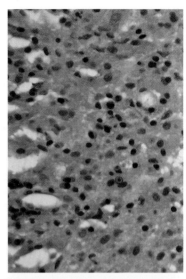

**Fig. 129** Bladder: malakoplakia. Characteristic Michaelis–Gutmann bodies. H&E.

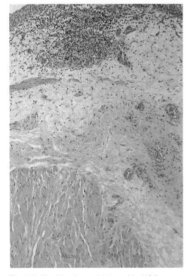

**Fig. 130** Bladder: Interstitial cystitis. H&E.

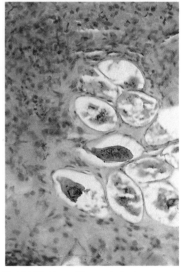

**Fig. 131** Bladder: schistosomiasis. Ova embedded in bladder wall. H&E ×40.

# 37 / Urinary tract tumours

Most urinary tract tumours arise in transitional epithelium; the majority occur in the bladder and have the potential to behave as malignant tumours. Transitional cell, squamous and adenocarcinomas are recognized. Transitional cell papilloma is a benign urothelial lesion.

*Aetiology*    Occupational exposure to β-naphthylamine and related compounds (azo dyes and pigments used in textile, printing, plastic, rubber and cable industries), smoking and abnormal tryptophan metabolism are implicated. Chronic vesical schistosomiasis is associated with the development of squamous cell carcinoma.

*Macroscopical*    Urinary tract tumours may have papillary or solid growth pattern (Figs 132 & 133). Invasion is more frequent in solid lesions. Flat plaques are also seen associated with in situ mucosal neoplasia.

*Microscopical*    **Transitional cell papilloma:** lesion composed of numerous finger like papillae, with central delicate fibrovascular core covered by no more than 5 layers of transitional cells.

**Transitional cell carcinoma:** papillary or solid lesions composed of transitional cells exhibiting varying grades of atypia, graded 1–3, with or without stromal invasion (Figs 134 & 135). About 70% are papillary, grade 1 and non-invasive.

**Squamous carcinoma** has no special features.

**Adenocarcinoma** arises in periurethral glands, cystitis cystica, urachal remnants or metaplastic mucosa. Mucin production may occur, including a rare signet-ring variant.

*Prognosis*    Determined by cell type, histological grade and stage of tumour. Staging is determined by depth of bladder wall invasion, extent of pelvic and lymph node spread and presence of distant metastases. There is a strong correlation between grade and stage.

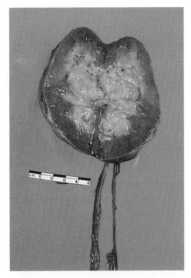

**Fig. 132** Transitional cell carcinoma of the renal pelvis.

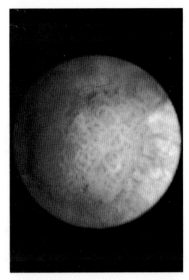

**Fig. 133** Bladder: cystoscopic view of a papillary tumour.

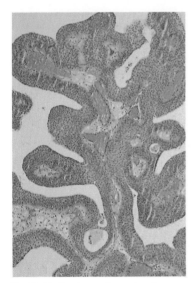

**Fig. 134** Bladder: low grade, non-invasive papillary transitional cell carcinoma. H&E ×40.

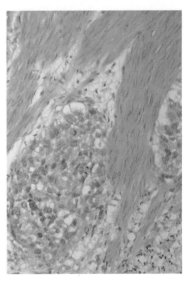

**Fig. 135** Bladder: high grade, solid, invasive transitional cell carcinoma. H&E ×40.

## Congenital

Epispadias (dorsal urethral opening) and hypospadias (ventral opening) may be associated with testicular maldescent. Phimosis interferes with cleanliness and may lead to paraphimosis (Fig. 136) and urethral obstruction.

## Inflammation

Specific inflammation is usually venereal, e.g. syphilis, gonorrhoea, chancroid, granuloma inguinale, herpes and condyloma acuminatum. Balanoposthitis is non-specific infection of the glans complicating phimosis or paraphimosis.

## Tumours

Over 95% are squamous carcinoma, with malignant melanoma next in frequency.

*Incidence* Age, 40–70 yrs; rare in UK but common in Africa, Asia and South America where it constitutes up to 10% of all cancers.

*Aetiology* Poor personal hygiene and presence of smegma bacillus may predispose as circumcision protects. Bowen's disease and erythroplasia of Queyrat are recognized premalignant disorders.

*Macroscopical* An ulcerating lesion at the coronal sulcus with irregular heaped-up margins, or a fungating papillary mass destroying the glans (Fig. 137).

*Microscopical* Often a poorly differentiated squamous carcinoma (Fig. 138). Invasion of the urethra or corpora cavernosum is a poor prognostic sign.

*Prognosis* Slowly growing, locally metastasizing tumour, but 25% have nodal deposits at presentation. If lesion limited to glans, 95% 5 yr survival, but with shaft or nodal involvement, this drops to 40%.

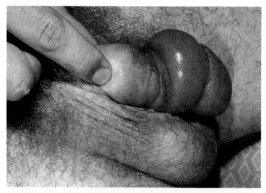

**Fig. 136** Penis: paraphimosis.

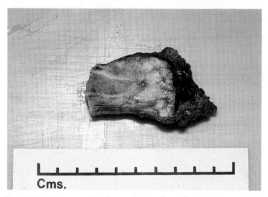

**Fig. 137** Penile amputation for carcinoma. Fungating tumour involving glans.

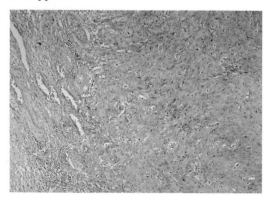

**Fig. 138** Penis: squamous carcinoma. H&E.

# 39 / **Testes**

## Cryptorchidism

*Definition*   Failure of testis to complete its normal descent.

*Incidence*   One or both testes are undescended at birth in 4% of full-term boys. By 1 yr, descent is complete in 75%. Of the rest, 70% are high scrotal, 20% inguinal and 10% intra-abdominal (Fig. 139).

*Aetiology*   Unknown, but possibilities include maternal hormonal withdrawal, intrauterine infection or congenital abnormality of the cord.

*Macroscopical*   Testis is smaller and softer than normal.

*Microscopical*   Little change up to 3 yrs but, later, tubular atrophy, peritubular fibrosis, prominent interstitial Leydig cells and foci of Sertoli cell hyperplasia (Fig. 140).

*Prognosis*   There is increased risk of torsion, trauma, infertility and tumour. Tumour risk is increased 30–50-fold, and greatest for intra-abdominal testes. About 10% of all testicular germ cell tumours arise in undescended testes. Early orchidopexy may preserve fertility, but tumour risk remains.

## Torsion

*Definition*   Twisting of spermatic cord resulting in testicular infarction and ischaemic atrophy.

*Aetiology*   Unduly long mesorchium, high insertion of tunica vaginalis, and maldescent predispose to torsion.

*Macroscopical*   Swollen, congested testis (Fig. 141).

*Microscopical*   Infarcted testis shows congestion, oedema and interstitial haemorrhage. After 8 h, irreversible tubular necrosis is seen, with later atrophy and interstitial fibrosis.

*Prognosis*   Early surgical correction may save testis.

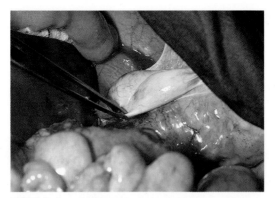

**Fig. 139** Undescended intra-abdominal testis.

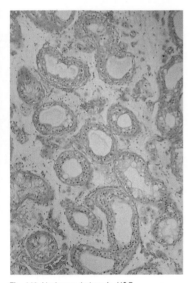

**Fig. 140** Undescended testis. H&E.

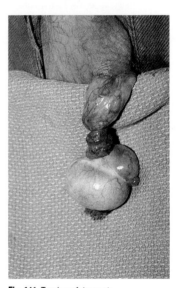

**Fig. 141** Torsion of the testis.

# 40 / Tumours of the testes

*Incidence*    Germ cell tumours are the commonest malignant tumours in men aged 25–35. Lymphomas and tumours of interstitial cells and appendages also seen.

## Seminoma

*Incidence*    Commonest testicular tumour, especially in cryptorchid testes. Peak incidence 30–40 yrs.

*Macroscopical*    Enlarged testis with solid lobulated pink/grey tumour (Fig. 142) and occasional yellow foci of necrosis.

*Microscopical*    Trabeculae or sheets of uniform round cells with clear cytoplasm, rounded nuclei with prominent nucleoli (Fig. 143). There is often interstitial lymphocyte infiltrate and syncytial or mulberry giant cells and/or a granulomatous reaction.

*Prognosis*    Depends on stage and presence of metastases. As tumour is radiosensitive and often presents early, overall survival is 90% at 5 yrs.

## Teratoma

*Incidence*    Peak incidence 20–30 yrs.

*Macroscopical*    Enlarged testis with whitish grey tumour with areas of necrosis, haemorrhage and cyst formation (Fig. 144).

*Microscopical*    **Teratoma differentiated (TD)** with mature well-differentiated ecto-, meso- and endoderm elements.
**Malignant teratoma intermediate (MTI)** with mixture of differentiated and embryonal tissue (Fig. 145).
**Malignant teratoma undifferentiated (MTU)** with entirely malignant tissue often anaplastic.
**Malignant teratoma trophoblastic (MTT)** with syncytio- and cytotrophoblast in villous form. Human chorionic gonadotrophin (HCG) is produced by trophoblast and those with yolk sac elements produce α-fetoprotein.

*Prognosis*    Less favourable. Depends on tumour subtype and stage. Chemotherapy is improving the outlook.

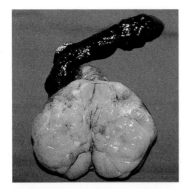

**Fig. 142** Testis: seminoma. Note uniform pale grey cut surface.

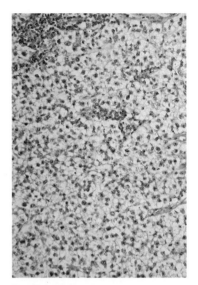

**Fig. 143** Testis: seminoma. H&E.

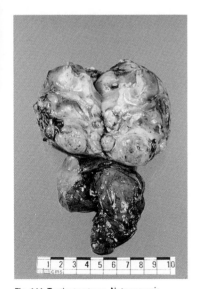

**Fig. 144** Testis: teratoma. Note necrosis, haemorrhage and cyst formation.

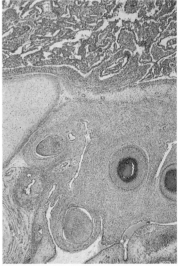

**Fig. 145** Testis: malignant teratoma intermediate. H&E.

# 41 / **Prostate**

## Benign prostatic hypertrophy (BPH)

*Incidence*    Common condition, increasing with age, so that 75% of men over age of 85 yrs have some degree of BPH.

*Aetiology*    Probable that the fall in androgen/oestrogen ratio with age stimulates overgrowth of the oestrogen dependent central prostatic glands.

*Macroscopical*    Firm nodular enlargement of lateral lobes and tissue posterior to the urethra (middle lobe).

*Microscopical*    Overgrowth of stromal and glandular elements with papilliferous ingrowths, adenoma-like nodules and focal cystic dilatation with concentric concretions (corpora amylacea). Stroma may form leiomyomatous nodules (Fig. 146).

*Prognosis*    Benign but produces bladder outlet obstruction.

## Carcinoma

*Incidence*    Fourth commonest cancer cause of death in men. Increases with age so that 90% of men over 90 yrs have histological identifiable foci of carcinoma.

*Aetiology*    Unknown, but possibly hormonal. No commoner in BPH than would be expected from age incidence.

*Macroscopical*    Irregular enlargement with hard white tissue.

*Microscopical*    Microacinar pattern of adenocarcinoma with small infiltrating glands (Fig. 147) and variable mucin production and perineural lymphatic permeation.

*Prognosis*    Depends on age, stage and histological grade. Many present with disseminated disease, especially sclerotic deposits in bone.

*Treatment*    Symptomatic control may be achieved by a combination of surgery, hormonal therapy (including orchidectomy) and irradiation.

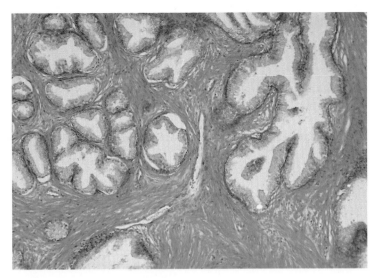

**Fig. 146** Benign prostatic hyperplasia. H&E.

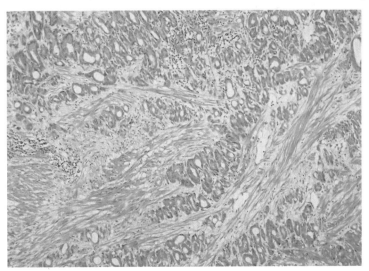

**Fig. 147** Adenocarcinoma of the prostate. Typical microacinar morphology. H&E.

# 42 / Inflammatory lesions of the breast

## Acute mastitis

*Aetiology*    Usually staphylococcal infection via nipple and ducts, often during lactation.

*Macroscopical*    Skin erythema with swelling and oedema of breast tissue (Fig. 148). Pus filled ducts or frank abscesses.

*Microscopical*    Acute inflammatory exudate involving ducts, with later periductal extension and abscess formation.

*Prognosis*    Untreated it causes abscesses, and scarring with nipple retraction that may mimic carcinoma.

## Fat necrosis

*Aetiology*    Usually a result of trauma to the breast.

*Macroscopical*    Central area of haemorrhage with oily fluid filled cavities surrounded by dense white calcified tissue and late fibrotic scarring.

*Microscopical*    Necrotic tissue replaced by acute inflammatory exudate, foamy lipid-laden macrophages, foreign body giant cells with cholesterol crystals, haemosiderin and granulation tissue (Fig. 149).

*Treatment*    Excision is curative and excludes malignancy.

## Duct ectasia

*Aetiology*    Inspissation of breast secretion, dilatation and rupture of ducts with inflammation. Commonest in non breast feeding multipara.

*Macroscopical*    Subareaolar ducts dilated with cheesy material.

*Microscopical*    Ducts containing acidophilic debris and foamy macrophages with ulceration and atrophy of epithelium. Chronic inflammatory infiltrate (Fig. 150) with plasma cells and foreign body giant cells.

*Prognosis*    Chronic nipple discharge, breast sepsis, mammary fistula and fibrosis if untreated.

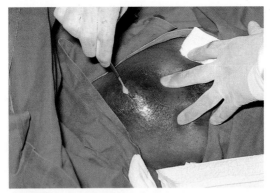

**Fig. 148** Breast: acute mastitis.

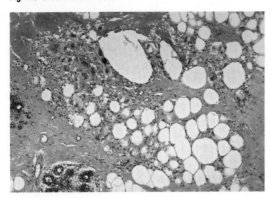

**Fig. 149** Breast: fat necrosis. H&E.

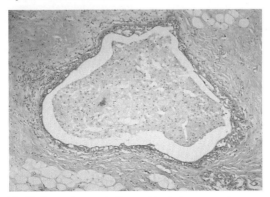

**Fig. 150** Breast: duct ectasia. Note periductal plasmacytic infiltrate. H&E.

# 43 / Fibrocystic disease of the breast (cystic mastopathy)

*Definition* Benign condition characterized by cyst formation, hyperplasia of duct epithelium (epitheliosis), enlargement of lobules (adenosis) and fibrosis.

*Incidence* Commonest disorder of female breast between puberty and menopause.

*Aetiology* Possibly the result of abnormal response to hormonal changes and can be associated with menstrual irregularities, nullipara and oestrogen administration.

*Macroscopical* Ill defined area of induration or firm swelling, often painful prior to menstruation. Cut surface shows variable fibrosis and cystic change.

*Microscopical* **Cysts** are localized dilatations of terminal ductules, lined by flattened epithelium, often with apocrine metaplasia (large columnar cells with eosinophilic cytoplasm) surrounded by myoepithelial cells (Fig. 151).

**Epitheliosis** may be solid or cribriform overgrowth of bland epithelial cells that overlap (Fig. 152). Lack of mitoses and necrosis help to distinguish it from carcinoma in situ.

**Adenosis** is a physiological process in pregnancy and secretory phase of menstrual cycle, persisting in fibrocystic disease. Sclerosing adenosis is characterized by disorderly proliferation of lobular epithelium and myoepithelium (Fig. 153) mimicking stromal invasion.

**Fibrosis** is variable and often only represents involutional change. Localized areas may present as distinct lumps (fibrous mastopathy) (Fig. 154).

*Prognosis* Cysts, apocrine metaplasia, adenosis and fibrosis are not associated with increased cancer risk. Epitheliosis increases risk twofold with strong family history of breast cancer.

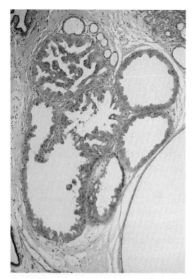

**Fig. 151** Breast: cystic apocrine metaplasia. H&E.

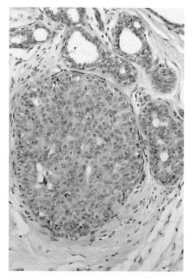

**Fig. 152** Breast: benign epitheliosis. H&E.

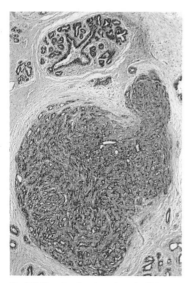

**Fig. 153** Breast: sclerosing adenosis. Note relationship to lobule. H&E.

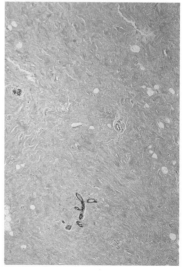

**Fig. 154** Breast: fibrous mastopathy. H&E.

# 44 / Benign tumours of the breast

## Fibroadenoma

*Definition*  Benign epithelial and stromal tumour occurring mainly in young women.

*Incidence*  Commonest benign breast tumour.

*Macroscopical*  Well-circumscribed, elastic round or ovoid mass with homogenous pale grey cut surface.

*Microscopical*  Two growth patterns are seen, pericanalicular, where lobular epithelial elements are surrounded by loose connective tissue (Fig. 155) and intracanalicular with curved and branching epithelial-lined clefts into which proliferating connective tissue appears to push (Fig. 156).

*Prognosis*  Excision is curative. Uncommonly, mesenchymal tumours can arise from the stroma, e.g. cystosarcoma phylloides, and very rarely lobular carcinoma from the epithelial component.

## Intraduct papilloma

*Definition*  Benign epithelial tumour arising from major ducts or lactiferous sinuses. It often causes nipple discharge or haemorrhage.

*Macroscopical*  Pedunculated, rounded or papillary tumour distending affected duct or sinus, often with macroscopical evidence of distal duct ectasia.

*Microscopical*  Composed of branching fibrovascular stroma covered by a double layer of outer cuboidal or columnar epithelium lying on myoepithelial cells (Fig. 157). Must be distinguished from papillary epitheliosis (no stromal core) or the much rarer papillary carcinoma (usually single layer of overtly malignant cells).

*Treatment*  Excision is curative.

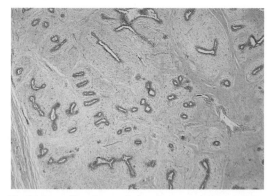

**Fig. 155** Breast: fibroadenoma. Pericanalicular growth pattern. H&E ×25.

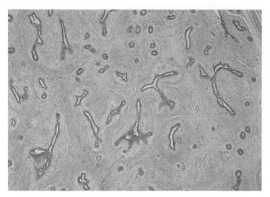

**Fig. 156** Breast: fibroadenoma. Intracanalicular growth pattern. H&E ×25.

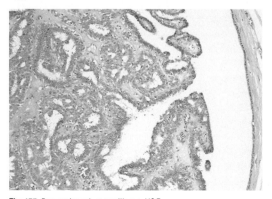

**Fig. 157** Breast: intraduct papilloma. H&E.

# 45 / **Carcinoma of the breast**

*Incidence*  Commonest malignant neoplasm in women in England and Wales (approximately 12 000 deaths/yr) representing 20% of cancer deaths in women. Annually, 86 new cases per 100 000 women/yr.

*Aetiology*  Risk is increased by early menarche, late menopause and strong family history, and reduced by oophorectomy and breast feeding. The role of the contraceptive pill is disputed.

## Ductal carcinoma

### Ductal carcinoma in situ
Accounts for 3–5% of breast cancers and presents as ill defined lump or incidental finding.

*Macroscopical*  Thick walled ducts with normal breast parenchyma. Squeezing ducts produces worm-like masses of tumour, 'comedo carcinoma'.

*Microscopical*  Dilated ducts filled with malignant cells growing in sheets or cribriform pattern or with central necrosis and foci of calcification (Fig. 158).

*Prognosis*  Multicentric in 33% and may be bilateral. Wide local excision gives good prognosis.

### Invasive ductal carcinoma
Accounts for 75% of all breast carcinomas.

*Macroscopical*  Irregular, spiky, grey-white tissue, cutting like unripe pear. May show yellow foci of elastosis (Fig. 159).

*Microscopical*  Spherical malignant cells with variable gland formation and mitoses set in a dense hyaline collagenous stroma (Fig. 160).

*Prognosis*  Depends on size of primary, extent of nodal involvement and histological differentiation. Overall 50% 5 yr survival.

### Paget's disease of the nipple
Weeping eczematous lesion of nipple and areola from extension of underlying intraduct carcinoma.

*Microscopical*  Malignant epithelial (Paget's) cells in lower epidermis with dermal inflammation and fibrosis (Fig. 161).

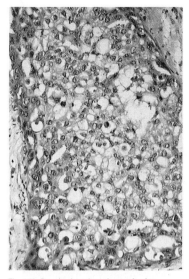

**Fig. 158** Breast: ductal carcinoma in situ. Compare with Figure 152. H&E.

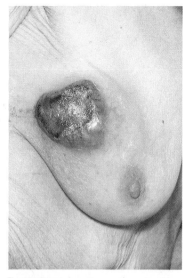

**Fig. 159** Breast: fungating carcinoma involving skin.

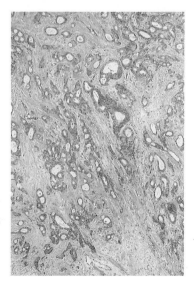

**Fig. 160** Breast: invasive ductal carcinoma. H&E.

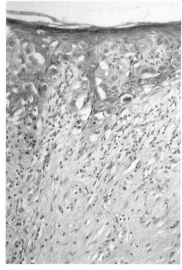

**Fig. 161** Breast: Paget's disease of the nipple. H&E.

## Lobular carcinoma

### Lobular carcinoma in situ

*Microscopical*    Distended lobules filled with uniform round cells with nuclei showing few atypical features (Fig. 162).

*Prognosis*    Frequently multicentric (60%) and associated with a significant risk of carcinoma in the ipsilateral and contralateral breast.

### Invasive lobular carcinoma
Accounts for 5–10% of all breast carcinomas.

*Macroscopical*    Often small, poorly defined, rubbery mass.

*Microscopical*    Small, uniform round neoplastic cells arranged in single 'Indian' file between collagen fibres and concentric rings about ducts (targetoid configuration) (Fig. 163).

*Prognosis*    Often bilateral (20%) and frequently multicentric. More often oestrogen receptor positive than is ductal carcinoma.

## Medullary carcinoma

*Macroscopical*    Large soft fleshy mass with foci of necrosis.

*Microscopical*    Sheets of large cells with pleomorphic vesicular nuclei and marked lymphoid infiltrate (Fig. 164).

*Prognosis*    Better than ductal carcinoma even with nodal metastases (84% 10 yr survival).

## Colloid (mucoid) carcinoma

*Macroscopical*    Large, soft, gelatinous, pale grey-blue mass.

*Microscopical*    Small islands of tumour cells floating in masses of pale blue staining amorphous mucin (Fig. 165).

*Prognosis*    Favourable, with lower incidence of nodal metastases (90% 10 yr survival).

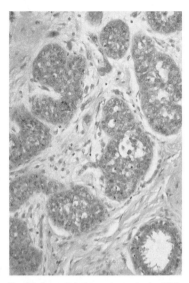

**Fig. 162** Breast: lobular carcinoma in situ. H&E.

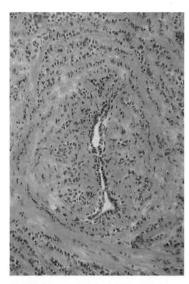

**Fig. 163** Breast: infiltrative lobular carcinoma. H&E.

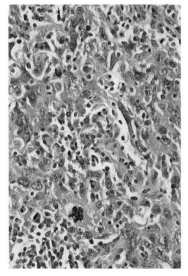

**Fig. 164** Breast: medullary carcinoma. H&E.

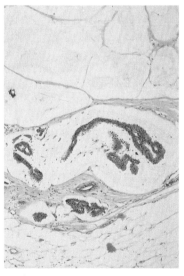

**Fig. 165** Breast: mucinous (colloid) carcinoma. H&E.

# 46 / Adrenal gland tumours

## Adrenocortical tumour (ACT)

*Incidence*  Small ACTs are incidental in 2–7% autopsies. Functioning or malignant ACTs are rare, but can produce Cushing's syndrome, precocious puberty in males or female virilization. Component of multiple endocrine adenoma (MEA) syndrome type I.

*Macroscopical*  Benign ACTs are well defined brown nodules, but aggressive ACTs are large and ill defined, with focally necrotic and haemorrhagic cut surface.

*Microscopical*  Varies from regular sheets of cells like zona fasciculata to anaplastic giant cell forms (Fig. 166).

## Phaeochromocytoma

*Incidence*  Rare tumour of chromaffin cells from the adrenal medulla. May be familial or associated with MEA type II or von Recklinghausen's disease. 10% are bilateral, 10% extra-adrenal and 10% malignant.

*Macroscopical*  Light brown, lobulated tumour (Fig. 167) turning brown-black in dichromate (chromaffin reaction).

*Microscopical*  Large polyhedral cells with copious granular basophilic cytoplasm in delicate vascular stroma (Fig. 168).

## Neuroblastoma

*Incidence*  Malignant tumour of neural crest derived cells. 80% occur under 5 yrs of age.

*Macroscopical*  Soft lobular haemorrhagic and necrotic tumour.

*Microscopical*  Small dark round or oval cells forming rosettes with central cytoplasmic fibrillary processes (Fig. 169). Occasionally partly calcified.

*Prognosis*  3 yr survival is 90% for stage I (limited to adrenal), but 2.5% for stage IV (distant spread).

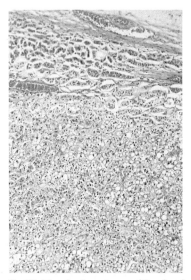

**Fig. 166** Adrenal: primary tumour of the adrenal cortex.

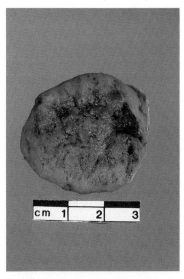

**Fig. 167** Adrenal: phaeochromocytoma.

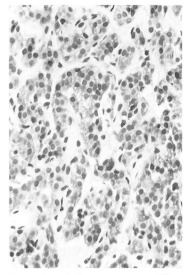

**Fig. 168** Adrenal: phaeochromocytoma. H&E ×40.

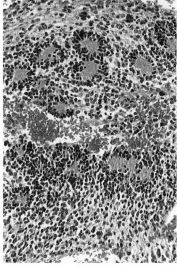

**Fig. 169** Adrenal: neuroblastoma. H&E ×40.

# 47 / **Non-toxic goitre**

*Definition*  Goitre means enlargement of the thyroid gland. Non-toxic, non-inflammatory goitres may be endemic in 'goitrous' areas or sporadic.

*Aetiology*  Non-toxic goitre results from compensatory hyperplasia following inadequate thyroxine production due to poor iodide intake or impaired enzyme activity. Endemic goitre occurs in remote areas (the Alps, Pyrenees, Himalayas, Derbyshire peaks), where local water is deficient in iodide. Sporadic goitre is due to dietary iodide deficiency, dyshormonogenesis or drugs that interfere with thyroxine synthesis.

*Macroscopical*  Non-toxic goitre is divided into parenchymatous and colloid varieties and both may be diffuse or nodular. Parenchymatous goitre shows gland enlargement and lack of translucency resembling pancreas. Colloid goitre has firm brown thyroid tissue (Fig. 170) with colloid accumulation. Areas of haemorrhage, fibrosis, calcification and cyst formation are common. Diffuse goitre affects the whole gland, while nodular goitre can be limited to one lobe.

*Microscopical*  **Parenchymatous goitre** shows enlargement of acinar cells to columnar type, with small, colloid deficient acini. Hyperplastic foci of this type enlarge, compressing adjacent glands to produce a nodular configuration (Fig. 171).

**Colloid goitre** shows enlarged distended acini, with deeply staining colloid and flattened epithelium. Foci of hyperplastic epithelium are often present between distended acini (Fig. 172).

*Behaviour*  Majority are euthyroid. Pressure effects may result from a greatly enlarged gland, retrosternal extension or haemorrhage into a cyst or colloid nodule.

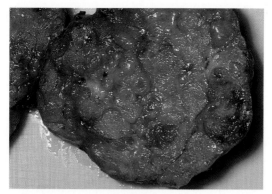

**Fig. 170** Thyroid: nodular colloid goitre.

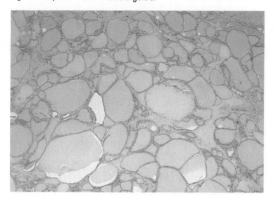

**Fig. 171** Thyroid: parenchymatous goitre. H&E ×25.

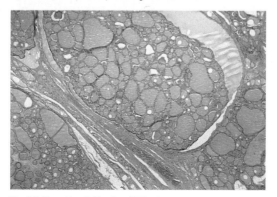

**Fig. 172** Thyroid: colloid goitre. H&E ×10.

## Hypothyroidism

*Definition*  Inadequate secretion of thyroxine, producing cretinism in infants and myxoedema in adults.

*Incidence*  Cretinism is now rare. Primary myxoedema is the most common variety of hypothyroidism. M:F = 1:5.

*Aetiology*  Cretinism may be endemic from iodide deficiency, or sporadic due to aplasia, hypoplasia or dyshormonogenesis. Myxoedema usually follows autoimmune chronic atrophic thyroiditis (1° myxoedema) or Hashimoto's disease, irradiation, dyshormonogenesis, hypopituitarism or resection.

*Macroscopical*  The gland is small, solid, pale and firm.

*Microscopical*  Gland is entirely replaced by hyaline fibrous tissue with lobular pattern and scattered small follicles lined by cells showing oxyphil metaplasia and islands of squamous metaplasia (Fig. 173) with a few lymphocytes and plasma cells.

## Hyperthyroidism

*Definition*  Overproduction of thyroxine usually due to Graves' disease. M:F, 1:5.

*Aetiology*  Primary hyperthyroidism (Graves' disease) (Fig. 174) is most often due to autoimmune thyroid stimulation by a long acting antibody reacting with TSH receptor. Rarely, it is due to autonomous hypersecretion by an adenoma or hyperfunctioning nodules developing in longstanding nodular colloid goitres.

*Macroscopical*  The gland is enlarged and often very vascular.

*Microscopical*  Acini of pale scalloped colloid, lined by hyperplastic columnar epithelium with papillary in-growths and a patchy lymphocyte infiltrate (Fig. 175). Appearances modified by prior medical treatment.

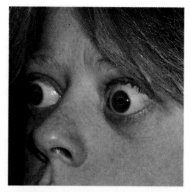

**Fig. 173** Thyroid: myxoedema. H&E ×25.

**Fig. 174** Thyroid: Graves' disease. Characteristic exophthalmos.

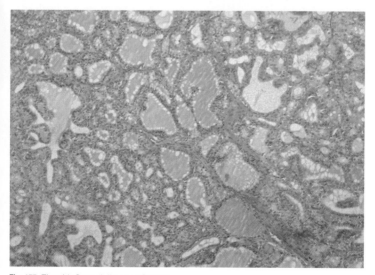

**Fig. 175** Thyroid: Graves' disease. H&E ×25.

# 49 / Thyroiditis

## Hashimoto's disease

*Incidence*    Commonest between 35 and 55 yrs. M:F = 1:12.

*Aetiology*    Autoantibodies against thyroglobulin and thyroid epithelial cell membrane are found in the serum. Patients tend to have higher incidence of auto-immune pernicious anaemia and Addison's disease.

*Macroscopical*    Firm, grey/white lobulated and distinct goitre (Fig. 176).

*Microscopical*    Diffuse interstitial lymphoid infiltrate with germinal centres, fibrosis and small acini with large acidophilic Hürthle/Askanazy cells (Fig. 177).

*Behaviour*    Hypothyroidism in 50% and may be associated with malignant lymphoma or papillary carcinoma.

## De Quervain's disease

*Definition*    Rare self-limiting thyroiditis. M:F = 1:2.

*Aetiology*    Probably response to viral infection or reactivation of latent virus.

*Macroscopical*    Indurated gland adherent to adjacent structures.

*Microscopical*    Necrotic follicles infiltrated by neutrophils, macrophages and epithelioid giant cells (Fig. 178).

## Riedel's thyroiditis

*Incidence*    Very rare. M:F = 1:4. Ages 35–55 yrs.

*Aetiology*    Unknown; can be associated with retroperitoneal fibrosis or end stage fibrotic Hashimoto's.

*Macroscopical*    Woody, hard, enlarged gland adherent to adjacent structures, often with tracheal compression.

*Microscopical*    Dense collagen and scattered compressed atrophic follicles and light inflammatory infiltrate (Fig. 179).

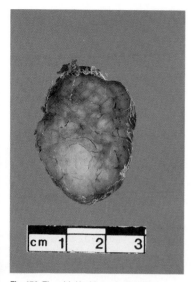

**Fig. 176** Thyroid: Hashimoto's disease.

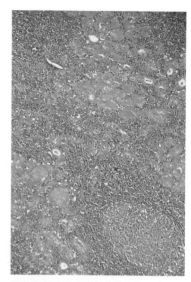

**Fig. 177** Thyroid: Hashimoto's. H&E ×25.

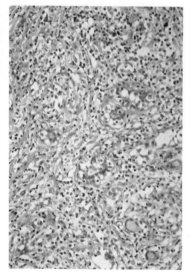

**Fig. 178** Thyroid: De Quervain's thyroiditis. H&E ×25.

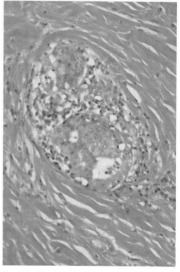

**Fig. 179** Thyroid: Riedel's thyroiditis. H&E ×25.

# 50 / Tumours of the thyroid

## Adenoma

*Definition*  Benign tumour of thyroid epithelium.

*Incidence*  Common; incidental finding in 10–21% autopsies.

*Macroscopical*  Solitary round or oval rubbery encapsulated lesion up to 8 cm diameter. Cut surface shows translucent brown or tan appearance (Fig. 180). Variable amount of necrosis, haemorrhage, fibrosis and calcification.

*Microscopical*  Mixture of large and small colloid follicles, small microfollicles and trabeculae of medium sized cells in interlacing alveolar network (Fig. 181). The fibrous capsule is intact, with no evidence of vascular invasion. Frequent foci of Hürthle cell metaplasia. Adenomas composed of large colloid follicles are difficult to differentiate from benign colloid nodules.

## Malignant tumours

*Introduction*  The vast majority are carcinomas derived from follicular epithelium, but lymphomas are also seen. There are two main categories of carcinoma: differentiated (papillary and follicular) and undifferentiated (anaplastic). A fourth variety, medullary carcinoma, is derived from C cells.

*Incidence*  Thyroid carcinoma accounts for 0.5% of all cancer deaths (400/yr). Commoner in women. Papillary carcinoma is commonest variety, especially in childhood and young adults.

*Aetiology*  Essentially unknown. Endemic goitre possibly associated with increase in follicular carcinoma, and thymic irradiation in childhood predisposes to papillary carcinoma. Some medullary carcinomas have familial incidence.

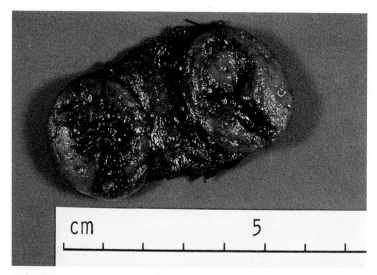

**Fig. 180** Thyroid: benign adenoma.

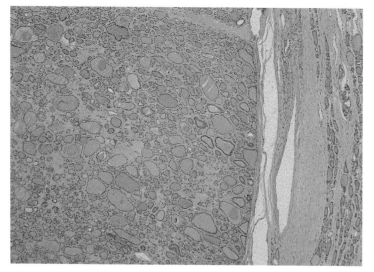

**Fig. 181** Thyroid: benign adenoma. Note uniform microfollicles and intact capsule. H&E ×10.

## Papillary carcinoma

*Macroscopical* Grey/white poorly defined nodule varying in size from a few millimetres to several centimetres. In large lesions haemorrhage, necrosis and cyst formation with visible papillae may be seen.

*Microscopical* Neoplastic epithelium on fibrovascular stalks often projecting into cystic spaces. Epithelium usually single layered and cuboidal with homogenous cytoplasm surrounding ovoid nucleus with fine chromatin and optically clear appearance ('Orphan Annie' nuclei) (Fig. 182). Laminated calcified spherules (psammoma bodies) are present in 40%.

*Prognosis* Slow growing and even with nodal metastases, survival may be prolonged. Overall 10 year survival is 84%, but with extrathyroid disease, it falls to 50%.

## Follicular carcinoma

*Macroscopical* Often indistinguishable from follicular adenoma as invasive nature only apparent histologically. Frankly invasive lesions are ill defined, fleshy, grey masses often with calcified fibrous centre and involvement of local structures (Fig. 183).

*Microscopical* Various sized follicles and/or trabecular cords of cuboidal neoplastic cells with compact hyperchromatic pleomorphic nuclei and scattered mitoses. Well differentiated tumours are only distinguished from adenomas by capsular or vascular invasion (Fig. 184). Hürthle cell carcinoma is a variant.

*Prognosis* Depends on extent of invasion and distant metastases. Spreads by bloodstream with lung and bone deposits. Overall 5 yr survival is 60%.

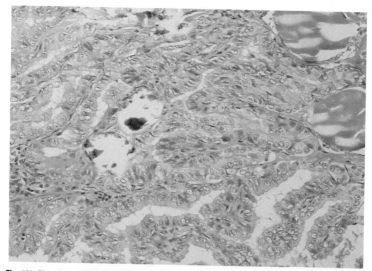

**Fig. 182** Thyroid: papillary carcinoma. Note clear nuclei and psammoma bodies. H&E ×25.

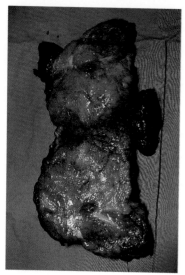

**Fig. 183** Thyroid: follicular carcinoma.

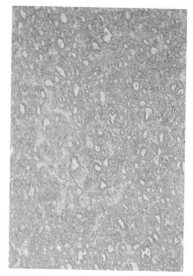

**Fig. 184** Thyroid: follicular carcinoma. H&E ×25.

## Undifferentiated (anaplastic) carcinoma

*Incidence*   10–15% of thyroid carcinomas, usually found in the elderly, presenting with rapid thyroid enlargement and respiratory distress. Surgery often followed by extensive local recurrence.

*Macroscopical*   Firm white tumour with necrosis, replacing thyroid and extending into adjacent structures.

*Microscopical*   Poorly differentiated tumours; three varieties seen:
- spindle cell tumour with cells in bundles or whorls resembling sarcoma with numerous mitoses (Fig. 185)
- small cell carcinoma consisting of round cells with hyperchromatic nuclei and scanty cytoplasm
- giant cell carcinoma with spindle cells and bizarre pleomorphic giant cells with frequent atypical mitoses (Fig. 186).

*Prognosis*   Poor. Overall 5 yr survival is 10–15%.

## Medullary carcinoma

*Definition*   Malignant tumour of parafollicular C cells.

*Incidence*   5–10% of thyroid tumours. M:F = 1:1. Usually over age of 40. Can be familial or part of MEA type II.

*Macroscopical*   Firm, grey, discrete, finely calcified mass and often multifocal. 50% have cervical nodal metastases at presentation.

*Microscopical*   Masses and nests of closely packed polygonal cells with eosinophilic granular cytoplasm and hyperchromatic nuclei set in hyaline fibrous stroma that stains for amyloid and may show calcium deposition (Fig. 187).

*Prognosis*   Protracted course, but dissemination by lymphatics and bloodstream is frequent. Overall 10 yr survival is 50%.

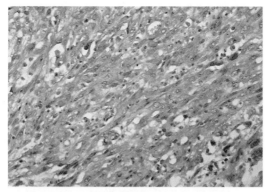

**Fig. 185** Thyroid: spindle cell anaplastic carcinoma. H&E ×40.

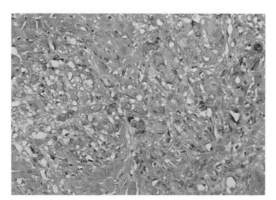

**Fig. 186** Thyroid: giant cell anaplastic carcinoma. H&E ×40.

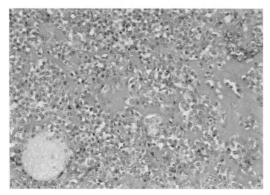

**Fig. 187** Thyroid: medullary carcinoma. H&E ×40.

# 51 / **Parathyroid glands**

## Hyperplasia

*Definition*   Primary or secondary (to hypocalcaemia) increase in constituent cells of all four glands.

*Incidence*   15% of all cases of primary hyperparathyroidism.

*Aetiology*   Unknown; chief cell hyperplasia found in MEA type I, occasionally in MEA II and may be familial.

*Macroscopical*   Enlarged and brown, the upper glands larger than lower ones in clear cell hyperplasia.

*Microscopical*   Clear cell hyperplasia has uniform appearance with large clear cells in solid masses or acini (Fig. 188). Chief cell hyperplasia has multiple nodules of chief cells mixed with oxyphil cells in solid, trabecular or follicular pattern devoid of fat.

## Adenoma

*Definition*   Benign tumour of parathyroid epithelial origin.

*Incidence*   80% of cases of primary hyperparathyroidism (HPT).

*Aetiology*   Unknown; in longstanding secondary hyperplasia one gland may become autonomous (tertiary HPT).

*Macroscopical*   Single, soft, well defined red/brown nodule (Fig. 189).

*Microscopical*   Solid sheets of chief, clear and oxyphil cells, with pleomorphic nuclei and variable size, but rim of normal parathyroid tissue (Fig. 190).

## Carcinoma

*Incidence*   Rare; 3% of cases of primary HPT.

*Macroscopical*   Firm irregular grey/white lobulated mass.

*Microscopical*   Pleomorphic cells with evidence of capsular or vascular invasion, often with nodal metastases.

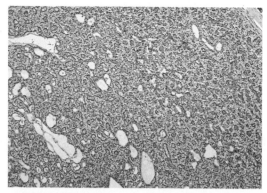

**Fig. 188** Parathyroid: diffuse hyperplasia. All four glands showed the same appearance. H&E ×25.

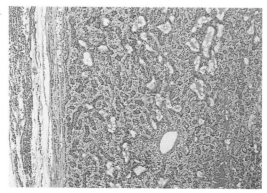

**Fig. 189** Parathyroid: adenoma—a single enlarged gland.

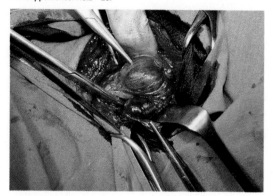

**Fig. 190** Parathyroid: adenoma. Note rim of normal parathyroid. H&E ×25.

### Seborrhoeic wart (seborrhoeic keratosis)

*Definition*   Benign tumour of epidermal basaloid cells.

*Incidence*   Very common in elderly, mainly trunk and face.

*Macroscopical*   Well demarcated, elevated, brown/black, often greasy, wart-like lesion of several centimetres (Fig. 191).

*Microscopical*   Thick interwoven tracts of basaloid cells with cystic inclusions of horny material (horn cysts). Hyperpigmentation is common (Fig. 192).

### Epidermal cyst

*Definition*   Benign intradermal lesion lined by stratified squamous epithelium and filled with keratin.

*Aetiology*   Most are spontaneous, but some arise from traumatic epidermal implantation.

*Macroscopical*   Slow growing, elevated, round intradermal or subcutaneous lesion on head, neck or trunk.

*Microscopical*   Cyst containing laminated keratin, surrounded by wall of true epidermis (Fig. 193). If it ruptures a florid foreign body giant cell reaction results.

### Pilar (trichilemmal) cyst

*Definition*   Benign cyst with keratinization analogous to outer root sheath of hair and epithelial lined.

*Incidence*   Common, but less so than epidermal cysts.

*Aetiology*   Unknown. Some inherited as autosomal dominant.

*Macroscopical*   Firm, smooth, white walled cyst on scalp in 90%.

*Microscopical*   Contains homogenous eosinophilic material and lined by squamous like epithelial cells without intracellular bridges, with nuclear palisading (Fig. 194).

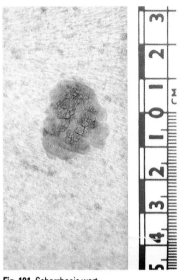

**Fig. 191** Seborrhoeic wart.

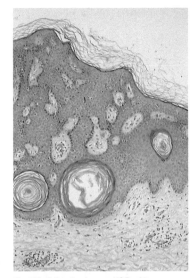

**Fig. 192** Seborrhoeic wart. H&E ×25.

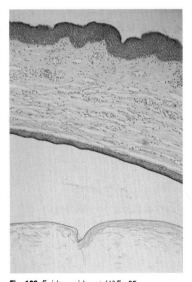

**Fig. 193** Epidermoid cyst. H&E ×25.

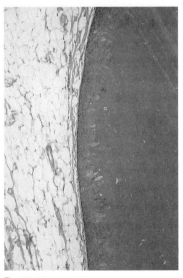

**Fig. 194** Pilar cyst. H&E ×25.

## Keratoacanthoma

*Definition*  Rapidly growing, self-limiting lesion of proliferating squamous epithelium with excess keratin filling a crater. Aetiology unknown.

*Incidence*  Relatively common, occurring in the elderly.

*Macroscopical*  Single firm dome shaped nodule, 1–2.5 cm, with a central horn-filled crater, usually occurring on exposed surfaces and occasionally multiple (Fig. 195).

*Microscopical*  Central, large, irregular, keratin filled crater lined by epidermis extending as a buttress over the sides. At the base irregular, interlacing, atypical epidermal proliferations, composed of glassy eosinophilic keratinizing squamous cells, extend into the dermis associated with a chronic inflammatory cell infiltrate (Fig. 196). Distinction from squamous cell carcinoma may be difficult without assessment of overall architecture.

## Adnexal tumours

**Pilomatrixoma** (calcifying epithelioma of Malherbe)

*Definition*  Benign tumour differentiating toward hair cells.

*Macroscopical*  Solitary firm nodule on upper body or face, often with red/blue discoloration of overlying skin.

*Microscopical*  Islands of basaloid cells merging with islands of 'ghost' cells. Calcification and foreign body giant cells often present (Fig. 197).

**Cylindroma**

*Definition*  Benign tumour differentiating to apocrine cells.

*Macroscopical*  Dome-shaped nodules on scalp. Multiple lesions in early adult life are dominantly inherited. May involve the entire scalp (turban tumour).

*Microscopical*  Lobulated tumour of irregular epithelial islands surrounded by hyaline membrane in loose stroma (Fig. 198).

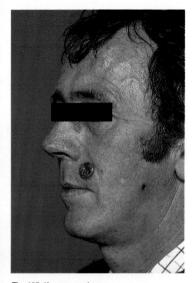

**Fig. 195** Keratoacanthoma.

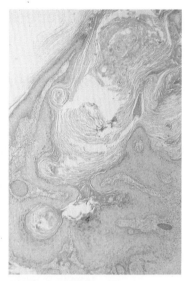

**Fig. 196** Keratoacanthoma. H&E ×25.

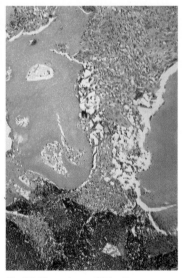

**Fig. 197** Pilomatrixoma. H&E ×40.

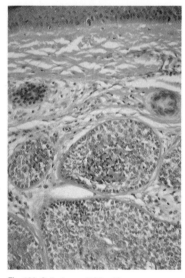

**Fig. 198** Cylindroma. H&E ×40.

# 53 / **Premalignant epidermal lesions**

## Solar keratosis

*Definition*  Common variety of squamous carcinoma-in-situ in sun exposed areas of fair skinned elderly adults.

*Aetiology*  Excessive exposure to sunlight over many years.

*Macroscopical*  Single/multiple dry scaly erythematous lesions, usually on face or back of hands. Some (Fig. 199) show marked hyperkeratosis and horn formation.

*Microscopical*  The epidermis shows hyperkeratosis with little or no parakeratosis (nuclei present in keratin layer), acanthosis (epidermal thickening) and dysplastic cells occupying most of the epidermis with basal layer crowding. In the dermis there is a dense chronic inflammatory infiltrate and collagen shows extensive basophilic degeneration (Fig. 200).

*Prognosis*  Squamous cell carcinoma may arise in up to 20%.

## Bowen's disease

*Definition*  Common variety of squamous cell carcinoma in situ involving whole thickness of epidermis.

*Aetiology*  Skin exposure to sunlight or arsenic ingestion.

*Macroscopical*  Irregular erythematous patch with sharp outline and scaling or crusting (Fig. 201). On the penis it is called erythroplasia of Queyrat.

*Microscopical*  Thickened epidermis with cells in disorder and large hyperchromatic nuclei, multipolar mitoses, bizarre multinucleate forms, parakeratosis and premature keratinization (dyskeratosis). The epidermodermal junction is sharp, with a chronic inflammatory infiltrate in the dermis (Fig. 202).

*Prognosis*  Squamous cell carcinoma develops in up to 10%.

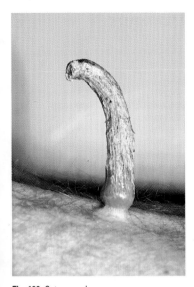

**Fig. 199** Cutaneous horn.

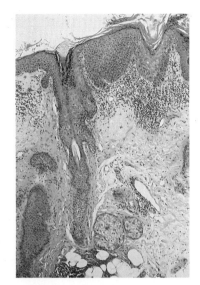

**Fig. 200** Solar keratosis. H&E ×40.

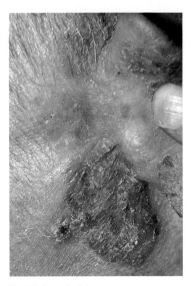

**Fig. 201** Bowen's disease.

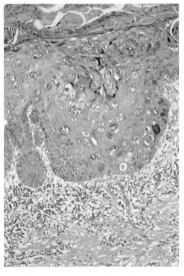

**Fig. 202** Bowen's disease. H&E ×40.

# 54 / Malignant epidermal tumours

## Squamous cell carcinoma

*Aetiology*  Most arise in sun damaged skin, in solar keratosis, or in chronic osteomyelitis (Marjolin's ulcer), burns scars, following irradiation or prolonged contact with hydrocarbons. Common in xeroderma pigmentosa.

*Macroscopical*  Shallow ulcer surrounded by wide, elevated, indurated border and frequently covered by a crust overlying a red granular base (Fig. 203).

*Microscopical*  A pleomorphic epithelial tumour with intercellular bridges and keratin formation (epithelial pearls) extending into the dermis or subcutis (Fig. 204). Poorly differentiated tumours may be difficult to identify as being squamous. Rare pseudoglandular and spindle cell variants are recognized.

*Prognosis*  Less than 2% metastasize to lymph nodes, but this occurs in up to 30% of those arising in scars.

## Basal cell carcinoma (BCC) (rodent ulcer)

*Aetiology*  Most occur on sun exposed skin, especially face, or after arsenic exposure. Occurs in two rare inherited disorders: basal cell naevus syndrome and xeroderma pigmentosa.

*Macroscopical*  Pearly grey, semitranslucent papule (Fig. 205) with telangiectasia and subsequent ulceration.

*Microscopical*  Dermal nests, cords and islands of round hyperchromatic cells with parallel elongation at the periphery (palisading) (Fig. 206). Variants include multicentric superficial keratinizing types, cystic or gland like (adenoid) forms and a morphoeic variant with dense dermal fibrosis.

*Prognosis*  May infiltrate deeply but rarely metastasize.

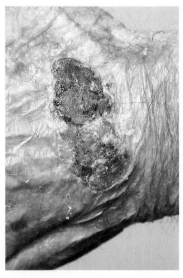

**Fig. 203** Squamous cell carcinoma on the back of the hand.

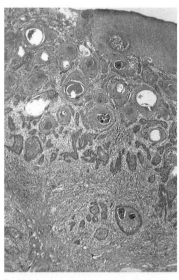

**Fig. 204** Squamous cell carcinoma. H&E ×10.

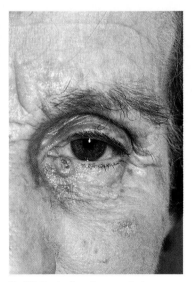

**Fig. 205** Basal cell carcinoma on the lower eyelid.

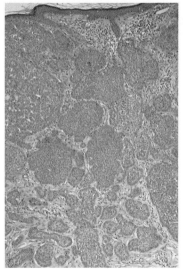

**Fig. 206** Basal cell carcinoma. H&E ×10.

# 55 / Benign pigmented naevi

| | |
|---|---|
| *Definition* | Benign tumours arising from neural crest derived cells that migrate to the epidermis in early fetal life. Such cells in the epidermis are called melanocytes and, if they migrate to the dermis (vide infra), naevus cells. |
| *Incidence* | Extremely common. Few individuals have none. |
| *Histogenesis* | Melanocytes normally lie among basal epidermal cells in the ratio 1:5 to 1:10. Most naevi begin in infancy as foci of melanocytic proliferation (junctional activity) in the epidermis and are termed junctional naevi. Later, melanocytes begin to grow into the dermis and the lesion with both intraepidermal and dermal components is called a compound naevus. Eventually the junctional component is lost and the naevus becomes exclusively dermal, an intradermal naevus. The process can be arrested at any stage. |
| *Macroscopical* | Junctional naevi are small, flat, brown/black lesions. Compound and intradermal naevi are similar, but usually elevated, occasionally hair bearing and papillomatous (Fig. 207). |
| *Microscopical* | Junctional naevi are composed of groups of melanocytes appearing as rounded cells with clear or eosinophilic cytoplasm with granular brown melanin pigmentation. Compound naevi (Fig. 208) show a similar pattern, but with naevus cells containing round or ovoid nuclei and scanty melanin, in the dermis. In intradermal naevi (Fig. 209), naevus cells are limited to the dermis and may be multinucleate. |
| *Prognosis* | Transformation to malignant melanoma is only a risk in naevi with junctional activity after puberty. 20% of malignant melanomas show evidence of a pre-existing benign naevus, but the overall risk of malignant change is small since pigmented naevi are very common and malignant melanoma is uncommon. |

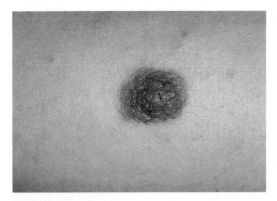

**Fig. 207** Benign naevus.

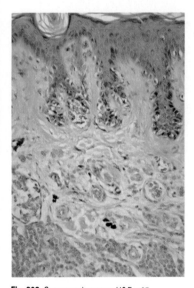

**Fig. 208** Compound naevus. H&E ×25.

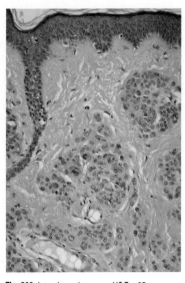

**Fig. 209** Intradermal naevus. H&E ×25.

# 56 / Malignant melanoma

| | |
|---|---|
| *Definition* | Malignant tumour of melanocytes with two principal types, superficial spreading and nodular melanoma, and two less common varieties, lentigo maligna and acral lentiginous melanoma. |
| *Incidence* | About 3:100 000 in England and Wales; 0.6% of all cancer deaths and rising. |
| *Aetiology* | Most arise de novo, although some occur in pre-existing naevi. Risk is increased in giant congenital naevi, dysplastic naevus syndrome and xeroderma pigmentosa. Sunlight with intermittent intense exposure is the most important factor. |
| *Macroscopical* | Superficial spreading presents as an irregular pigmented plaque with variable pigmentation usually on lower legs, chest or back (Fig. 210). Nodular melanoma (Fig. 211) presents as elevated dark nodule at any site. Lentigo maligna is a flat, slowly growing lesion on exposed skin of the elderly, while acral lentiginous melanomas occur on palms or soles in Africans or Orientals. |
| *Microscopical* | In each subtype malignant melanocytes are seen with abundant pink granular cytoplasm, highly pleomorphic nuclei and prominent nucleoli. Superficial spreading melanoma shows vertical dermal invasion and horizontal intraepidermal spread, extending for three or more rete ridges lateral to the edge of the vertical component (Fig. 212). Nodular melanoma by contrast has no significant horizontal intraepidermal component (Fig. 213). Lentigo maligna shows dysplastic melanocytes in linear growth along the basal epidermal layer, often with atrophic epidermis and solar collagen damage of the dermis. In some cases invasion of the dermis occurs. |
| *Prognosis* | Depends on depth of invasion (Clarke levels) and thickness of tumour, site, type of melanoma, mitotic rate, lymphocyte response, patient sex and presence of metastases, nodal or systemic. |

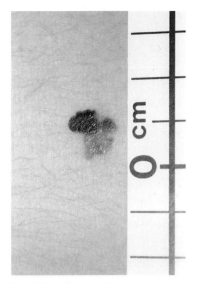

**Fig. 210** Superficial spreading malignant melanoma.

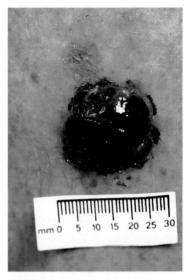

**Fig. 211** Nodular malignant melanoma.

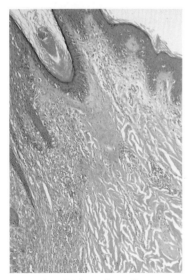

**Fig. 212** Superficial spreading malignant melanoma. H&E ×25.

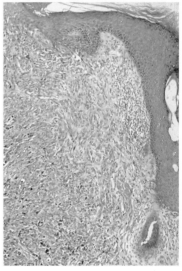

**Fig. 213** Nodular malignant melanoma. H&E ×25.

# 57 / **Dermal tumours**

## Dermatofibroma

*Definition*    Common elevated benign nodular proliferation of fibroblasts and histiocytes, often in lower limb.

*Aetiology*    About 20% have preceding trauma, suggesting that it may represent a proliferative response.

*Microscopical*    Interlacing pattern of collagen, fibroblasts, thin walled blood vessels, lipid or haemosiderin laden macrophages and giant cells (Fig. 214).

## Cutaneous fibrous polyp (skin tag)

*Macroscopical*    Common, soft, wrinkled, polypoid lesion.

*Microscopical*    Central core of fibrous tissue and fat covered by normal dermis (Fig. 215).

## Haemangioma

*Definition*    Common hamartomatous malformations. Multiple when associated with hereditary telangiectasia or Sturge-Weber syndrome.

*Macroscopical*    Well defined, small, deep red, elevated lesions, but may be large as facial 'port wine stains'.

*Microscopical*    Capillary lesions consist of networks of capillary vessels in the dermis with supplying artery, and cavernous lesions are composed of large interlacing vascular spaces (Fig. 216).

## Pyogenic granuloma

*Definition*    Common particular variety of haemangioma, probably a response to inflammatory stimulus.

*Microscopical*    Capillary vessels set in an oedematous stroma containing numerous polymorphs (Fig. 217).

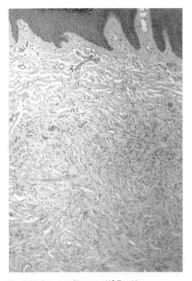

**Fig. 214** Dermatofibroma. H&E ×40.

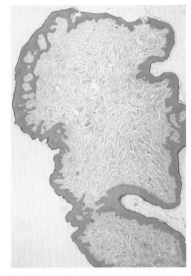

**Fig. 215** Fibroepithelial polyp (skin tag). H&E ×10.

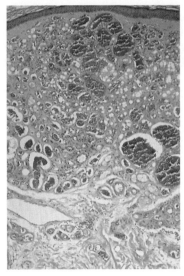

**Fig. 216** Benign capillary haemangioma. H&E ×10.

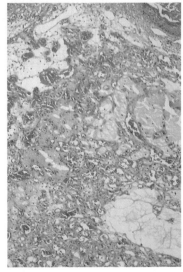

**Fig. 217** Pyogenic granuloma. H&E ×25.

## Lipoma

*Definition*      Common benign tumour of fat (Fig. 218).

*Macroscopical*      Single or multiple, well defined, lobulated, yellow masses of adipose tissue; may occur anywhere.

*Microscopical*      Mass of large, variably sized fat cells surrounded by thin fibrous capsule. Variants contain fibrous tissue (fibrolipoma) or vascular tissue (angiolipoma).

## Neurofibroma and neurilemmoma (Schwannoma)

*Definition*      Benign Schwann cell tumours of nerve roots or peripheral nerves, thus presenting in the dermis.

*Incidence*      Not uncommon, but in von Recklinghausen's disease multiple lesions of both type of tumour are seen.

*Macroscopical*      Solitary or multiple intradermal or subcutaneous nodules of varying size. A neurofibroma produces a fusiform swelling of the nerve, but a neurilemmoma displaces the nerve fibres which are spread over the surface of the lesion. A neurilemmoma is often partly cystic.

*Microscopical*      **Neurofibroma** consists of dense hyaline connective tissue mixed with elongated spindle shaped cells and residual nerve fibres (Fig. 219).

     **Neurilemmoma** consists of whorls and bundles of densely packed spindle cells arranged in parallel so that the nuclei form palisades (Antoni A tissue), intermixed with hypocellular loose pale staining tissue showing foci of cystic change (Antoni B tissue) (Fig. 220). Nerve fibres are not found in the tumour.

*Prognosis*      Excision is curative. Malignant change is a recognized complication in von Recklinghausen's disease (Fig. 221).

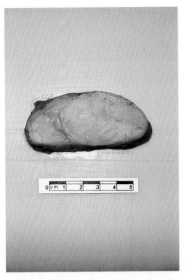

Fig. 218 Benign lipoma removed from the thigh.

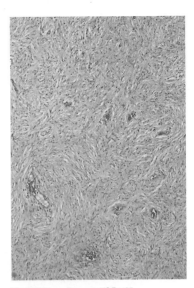

Fig. 219 Neurofibroma. H&E ×25.

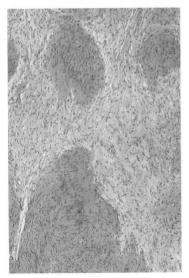

Fig. 220 Neurilemmoma. H&E ×25.

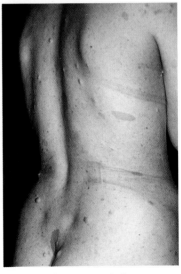

Fig. 221 Von Recklinghausen's disease (multiple neurofibromatosis).

## Viral warts (verrucae)

*Definition* Very common hyperplastic epidermal lesions caused by human papilloma virus.

*Macroscopical* Verruca vulgaris (common wart) is pale elevated lesion covered by horny skin. Verruca plana is a slightly elevated, flat, tan lesion on face or hands, while verruca plantaris or palmaris are hyperkeratotic lesions on sole or palm.

*Microscopical* Verruca vulgaris shows hyperkeratosis and papillomatosis with elongation and inbending of rete ridges. Large vacuolated cells are found in upper epidermis with eosinophilic cytoplasmic inclusions and basophilic nuclear inclusions (Fig. 222). Verruca plantaris (Fig. 223) shows marked hyperkeratosis and parakeratosis while v. plana has more thickened epidermis than papillomatosis.

## Condyloma acuminatum (venereal wart)

*Macroscopical* Soft tan, raspberry or cauliflower like viral wart limited to anogenital area.

*Microscopical* Thickened epidermis with elongated broad rete ridges containing vacuolated cells over loose supporting tissue with chronic inflammatory infiltrate. Mitoses frequent in epidermis.

## Molluscum contagiosum

*Definition* Specific viral lesion caused by a pox virus.

*Macroscopical* Multiple discrete skin coloured papules with central depression containing cheesy material.

*Microscopical* Cup shaped depressed epidermal proliferation with intracellular eosinophilic aggregates of cytoplasmic viral inclusions (molluscum bodies) (Fig. 224).

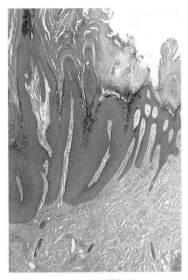

**Fig. 222** Verruca vulgaris. H&E ×25.

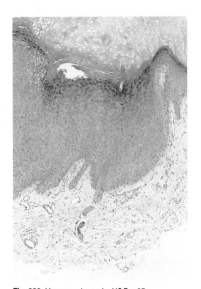

**Fig. 223** Verruca plantaris. H&E ×25.

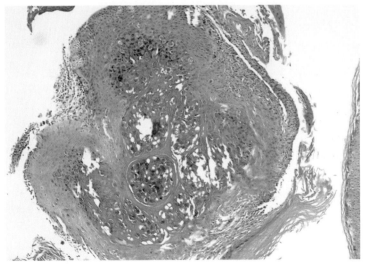

**Fig. 224** Molluscum contagiosum. H&E ×25.

# 59 / Malignant soft tissue tumours

### Malignant fibrous histiocytoma

*Nature*  Possibly of histiocytic or fibroblastic origin, occurring in lower limb, upper limb or abdominal cavity in relation to skeletal muscle or fascia.

*Microscopical*  Storiform (cartwheel like) pattern of plump fibroblasts mixed with histiocytes and variable multinucleate giant cells (Fig. 225). 50% 3 yr survival.

### Liposarcoma

*Nature*  Malignant tumour of adipose tissue, typically occurring in thigh, buttock and retroperitoneum; the most common malignant soft tissue tumour.

*Microscopical*  A variable mixture of adipocytes with primitive mesenchymal cells, ground substance and pleomorphic lipoblasts with minute fat vacuoles (Fig. 226).

### Leiomyosarcoma

*Nature*  Malignant tumour of smooth muscle typically occurring in the uterus or stomach, but occasionally arising from the media of blood vessels.

*Microscopical*  Interlacing bundles of plump smooth muscle cells with frequent mitoses, myofibrils and typical blunt ended nuclei (Fig. 227). 40% 5 yr survival.

### Fibrosarcoma

*Nature*  Malignant tumour of fibrous tissue arising from fascia and deep connective tissue at any site.

*Microscopical*  Interlacing bundles of spindle shaped fibroblasts with variable amounts of collagen; in better differentiated cases the cells are arranged in a 'herring-bone' pattern. Locally recurrent.

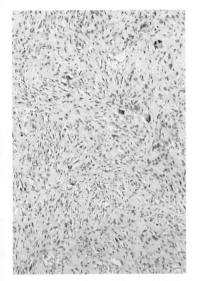

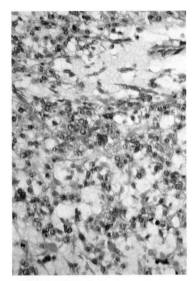

**Fig. 225** Malignant fibrous histiocytoma. H&E
×25.

**Fig. 226** Liposarcoma. Retroperitoneal tumour
in 70 yr old man. H&E ×25.

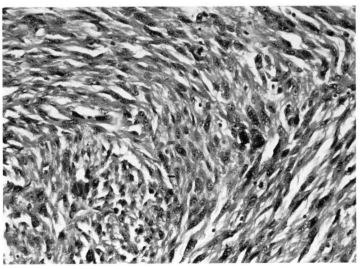

**Fig. 227** Leiomyosarcoma. H&E ×25.

## Vulval dystrophies

*Definition*   Heterogenous group of pale grey or white, opaque, plaque-like mucosal thickenings. Three types are seen: lichen sclerosus et atrophicus (LSA), hyperplastic dystrophy and a mixture of both.

*Incidence*   Most common age: 45–55 yrs.

*Microscopical*   LSA is characterized by epidermal atrophy, loss of rete pegs and replacement of dermis by dense collagenous fibrous tissue with bandlike chronic inflammatory infiltrate (Fig. 228). Hyperplastic dystrophy shows epithelial hyperplasia and hyperkeratosis with varying degrees of atypia up to carcinoma in situ (Fig. 229).

*Prognosis*   Hyperplastic dystrophy with atypia progresses to invasive carcinoma in 1–5%; LSA rarely does so.

## Vulval tumours

Benign tumours are rare; most malignant tumours are squamous carcinoma (SCC) (Fig. 230), malignant melanoma and basal cell carcinoma; carcinoma of Bartholins or sweat glands rarely occur.

*Incidence*   3% of female genital cancer; rare below 60 yrs.

*Aetiology*   SCC may be associated with vulval dystrophy, and has been associated with herpes simplex type II. Condylomas may coexist with atypia or carcinoma-in-situ, suggesting a possible viral aetiology.

*Macroscopical*   Firm, indurated, ulcerated lesion of the vulva.

*Microscopical*   Usually well or moderately differentiated squamous carcinoma as elsewhere in body (Fig. 231).

*Prognosis*   2 cm lesions without nodal involvement, 60–80% survival at 5 yrs. 65% have node involvement, first to inguinal, then pelvic, peri-rectal, iliac and para-aortic nodes.

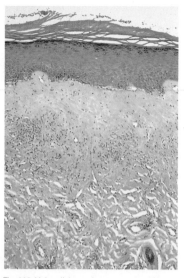

**Fig. 228** Vulva: lichen sclerosus et atrophicus. H&E ×25.

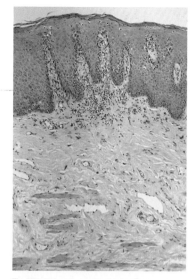

**Fig. 229** Vulva: hyperplastic vulval dystrophy. H&E ×25.

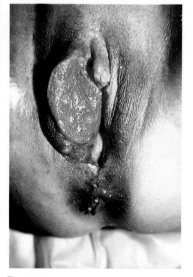

**Fig. 230** Vulva: squamous carcinoma.

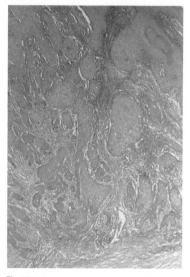

**Fig. 231** Vulva: squamous carcinoma. H&E ×10.

# 61 / **The cervix**

*Introduction*   Although cervical inflammation is common and benign tumours can occur, carcinoma is by far the most important cervical lesion.

## Cervical carcinoma

*Definition*   A malignant tumour of cervical epithelium. Squamous carcinoma accounts for 80% and adenocarcinoma the remainder.

*Incidence*   Approximately 2000 deaths/yr, equivalent to 3% of cancer deaths in women. 7th commonest cancer in women, with peak incidence at 45–55 yrs.

*Aetiology*   Epidemiological studies indicate cervical cancer is related to early onset of coitus and multiple sexual partners, suggesting venereal transmission of carcinogenic infectious agent. Human papilloma virus currently under suspicion.

*Natural history*   Cervical carcinoma evolves over 10–15 yrs from epithelium showing progressive degrees of cytological abnormality (dysplasia, intra-epithelial neoplasia). Such abnormal cells may be detected by exfoliative cytology, forming the basis for screening programmes.

*Macroscopical*   Cervical intraepithelial neoplasia (CIN) (Fig. 232) is identified at colposcopy or by the Schiller test. Invasive carcinoma presents as exophytic, friable, polypoid mass or endophytic ulcerated nodular mass (Fig. 233). Early spread to nodes.

*Microscopical*   CIN shows loss of maturation and polarity, with excess mitotic activity, increased nucleo-cytoplasmic ratio and pleomorphism (Fig. 234). Invasive carcinoma is most often squamous and similar to lesions elsewhere (Fig. 235).

*Prognosis*   Depends on stage. Stage 0 (CIN) 100% survival at 5 yrs, stage I (limited to cervix) 90% and stage IV (extension to pelvis, rectum, bladder) 10%.

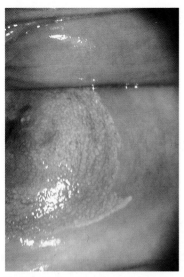

Fig. 232 Colposcopic appearance of CIN 3.

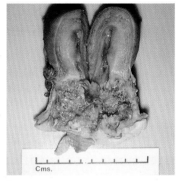

Fig. 233 Carcinoma of the cervix.

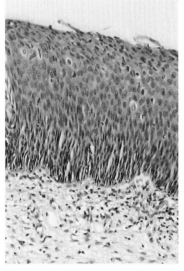

Fig. 234 Cervical intraepithelial neoplasia grade 3 (CIN 3) (carcinoma-in-situ). H&E ×40.

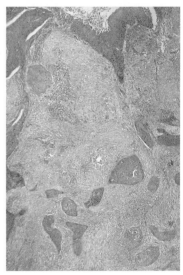

Fig. 235 Squamous cell carcinoma of cervix. H&E ×25.

## Endometrial hyperplasia

*Definition*  Excessive proliferation of endometrial glands and stroma which may be associated with a risk of developing endometrial adenocarcinoma.

*Aetiology*  Prolonged high oestrogen stimulation with minimal progesterone, e.g. anovulatory cycles, granulosa and theca cell tumours, excess adrenocortical activity, exogenous oestrogen.

*Macroscopical*  Large uterus; thick, polypoid, velvety endometrium.

*Microscopical*  **Cystic glandular hyperplasia** shows cystic change of hyperplastic glands in dense stroma (Fig. 236).
**Atypical hyperplasia** (Fig. 237) shows variable architectural and cytological atypia of glands.

*Prognosis*  Up to 50% of untreated *atypical hyperplasia* go malignant.

## Endometrial carcinoma

*Incidence*  10% of cancer in women, especially in postmenopausal nulliparous women age 55–65 yrs.

*Aetiology*  Abnormal prolonged oestrogen stimulation and often preceded by atypical hyperplasia.

*Macroscopical*  Localized polyp in fundus or diffuse tumour with large uterus, ulceration and bleeding (Fig. 238).

*Microscopical*  85% are adenocarcinomas with malignant endometrial glands (Fig. 239). 10–15% show foci of squamous differentiation, ranging from benign metaplasia to malignant cells. Rare clear cell, secretory, papillary serous and mucinous variants are seen.

*Prognosis*  Depends on stage and grade. Stage I (corpus only) 90% survival at 5 years, stage IV (beyond pelvis to rectum or bladder) 20%. Overall 60% at 5 yrs.

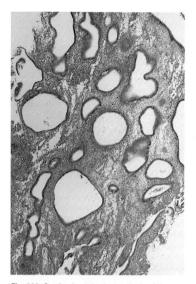

**Fig. 236** Cystic glandular hyperplasia of the endometrium. H&E ×25.

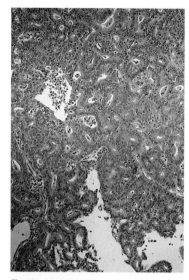

**Fig. 237** Atypical endometrial hyperplasia. H&E ×25.

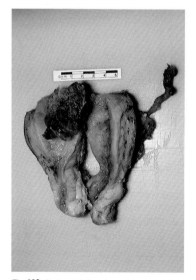

**Fig. 238** Endometrial carcinoma.

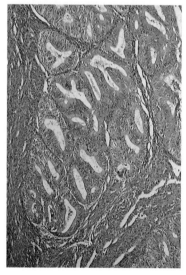

**Fig. 239** Endometrial adenocarcinoma. H&E ×25.

# 63 / **Myometrium**

## Tumours of the myometrium

*Incidence*  Benign leiomyomas (fibroids) arising from smooth muscle are the commonest tumour in women seen in 25% of women between 20–40 yrs. Sarcoma is rare.

*Macroscopical*  Often multiple encapsulated round firm masses embedded in myometrium (intramural), projecting beneath serosa (subserosal) or endometrium (submucosal). May become pedunculated (Fig. 240).

*Microscopical*  Interlacing bundles of smooth muscle in whorls and twists, with pale eosinophilic cytoplasm and elongated nuclei (Fig. 241). Degeneration seen as fibrosis, calcification, hyaline or fatty change.

*Prognosis*  Most asymptomatic; malignancy rare. Removed for pressure effects or menstrual irregularities.

## Endometriosis

*Definition*  Tissue histologically identical to endometrium found in distant sites, e.g. ovaries, fallopian tube, uterine ligaments, bowel, skin and lung.

*Incidence*  Peak 20–40 yrs, highest in social classes I and II.

*Aetiology*  Three theories: coelomic epithelial metaplasia; retrograde implantation of endometrium via tubes at menstruation; haematogenous spread.

*Macroscopical*  Red/blue nodules in affected organs that undergo cyclical change with periodic bleeding forming cystic areas with altered blood (chocolate cysts) (Fig. 242). Old lesions may be yellow/brown and cause fibrosis, distortion and adhesions.

*Microscopical*  Diagnosis requires presence of endometrial glands and stroma (Fig. 243). Old lesions may only have fibrosis and haemosiderin-laden macrophages.

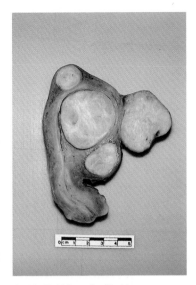

**Fig. 240** Multiple uterine fibroids.

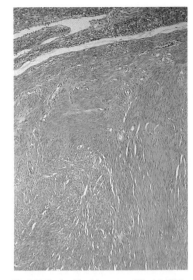

**Fig. 241** Benign fibroleiomyoma (fibroid). H&E ×25.

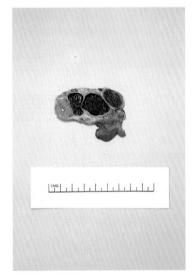

**Fig. 242** Endometriosis.

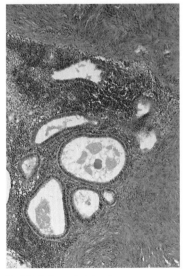

**Fig. 243** Endometriosis in a Caesarean scar. H&E ×25.

## Salpingitis

*Aetiology*    Most cases result from ascending infection via uterine cavity and can follow abortion, parturition, instrumentation and venereal disease, especially gonorrhoea, chlamydia and herpes virus. Patients with an IUCD have higher incidence, but many cases occur with no predisposing cause when organisms may be gram-positive cocci, coliforms or anaerobes.

*Macroscopical*    The tube is congested, swollen and tense with pus which may discharge from fimbrial end. Complications include tubo-ovarian abscess, fusion of fimbrial end with collection of clear fluid (hydrosalpinx) or pus (pyosalpinx), or chronic inflammation predisposing to infertility and ectopic pregnancy.

*Microscopical*    Features of non-specific inflammation with adhesion of fimbriae and plicae.

## Ectopic pregnancy

*Definition*    Implantation of fertilized ovum in any site other than uterus. 95% are in the fallopian tubes.

*Incidence*    1 in every 150 pregnancies.

*Aetiology*    About 50% occur in apparently normal tubes. Chronic salpingitis, previous tubal surgery, peritubal adhesions from appendicitis or endometriosis, an IUCD and tubal tumours or cysts predispose.

*Macroscopical*    Dilated tube filled with blood clot and placental tissue. Many cases rupture with intraperitoneal haemorrhage; some abort and resolve spontaneously.

*Microscopical*    Poorly developed decidual change and implanting placental villi in the tube wall (Fig. 244).

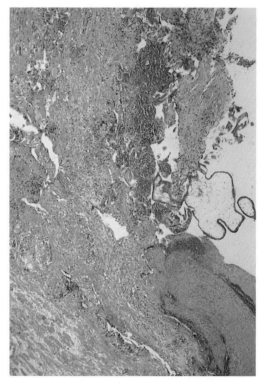

**Fig. 244** Fallopian tube ectopic pregnancy. Note implanted chorionic villi. H&E ×10.

# 65 / **Ovaries**

## Non-neoplastic cysts

*Definition*    Cysts from graafian follicles or corpora lutea.

*Incidence*    Very common (Fig. 245).

*Aetiology*    Follicular cysts arise from graafian follicles or sealed ruptured follicles. Luteal cysts arise from sealing of a haemorrhagic corpus luteum.

*Macroscopical*    Follicular cysts are usually multiple, in the cortex and filled with clear serous fluid. Luteal cysts are solitary, up to 3 cm and filled with amber fluid or altered blood.

*Microscopical*    Follicular cysts are lined by atrophic granulosa cells. Luteal cysts are lined by luteinized granulosa and theca cells (Fig. 246).

*Prognosis*    Usually innocuous but luteal cysts may rupture and bleed. Rarely, oestrogen production results in endometrial hyperplasia. Multiple follicular cysts occur in Stein-Leventhal syndrome.

## Germ cell tumours

*Incidence*    15–20% of ovarian tumours, the majority (95%) being benign cystic teratomas, seen between 20 and 30 yrs of age. Malignant forms, e.g. dysgerminoma (analogous to testicular seminoma), yolk sac and trophoblastic tumours are recognized.

*Macroscopical*    ***Benign cystic teratoma*** is usually a unilocular cyst containing sebaceous material and hair and lined by rough grey tissue resembling skin, with calcification and tooth structures (Fig. 247).

*Microscopical*    Cyst wall composed of stratified squamous epithelium with sebaceous glands, hair shafts and adnexal structures with other endodermal and mesodermal tissues such as bone, muscle, and gastrointestinal epithelium (Fig. 248).

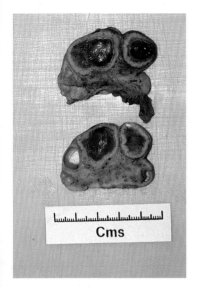

Fig. 245 Ovary: follicular and luteal cysts.

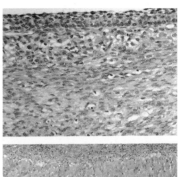

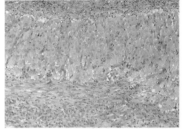

Fig. 246 Ovary: wall of adjacent follicular (above) and luteal (below) cysts. H&E ×40.

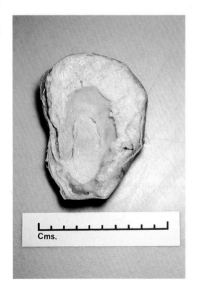

Fig. 247 Ovary: dermoid cyst (benign cystic teratoma).

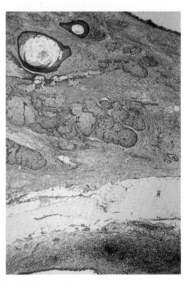

Fig. 248 Ovary: dermoid cyst. Note mature elements of all three germ cell layers. H&E ×10.

## Tumours of surface epithelium

*Introduction*  There are three types:
- *serous* (resembling fallopian tube)
- *mucinous* (resembling endocervical epithelium)
- *endometrioid* (resembling endometrium).

These are often cystic in benign, malignant or borderline forms, and termed cystadenoma or cystadenocarcinoma.

*Incidence*  75% of ovarian tumours. Third commonest female tumour; 3500 deaths yr. Serous tumours (30%) are seen between 20 and 50 yrs and are more often malignant than mucinous tumours (20%) which occur between 30 and 50 yrs; endometrioid forms (15–20%) are mainly malignant.

*Macroscopical*  **Serous** forms are ovoid, single or multilocular cysts, up to 40 cm, containing clear fluid. Cystadenomas have smooth lining; irregularity, nodularity and capsular penetration suggest malignancy. They are often bilateral (Fig. 249).

**Mucinous** tumours are filled with gelatinous fluid and can reach giant proportions (Fig. 250).

**Endometrioid** forms have solid and cystic areas with polypoid masses or papillae.

*Microscopical*  **Benign serous** tumours lined by single layer of tall columnar ciliated epithelium with papillae on a fibrovascular core. Malignant features include loss of nuclear polarity, multilayering solid epithelial masses and capsular or cyst wall invasion (Fig. 251).

**Mucinous** tumours are lined by columnar epithelium with mucinous vacuolation and absent cilia. Malignant features are as above.

**Endometrioid** ovarian carcinoma show features resembling typical endometrial adenocarcinoma.

*Prognosis*  Excision of cystadenomas is curative. 10 yr survival for cystadenocarcinomas is 15% for serous, 35% for mucinous and 40% for endometrial.

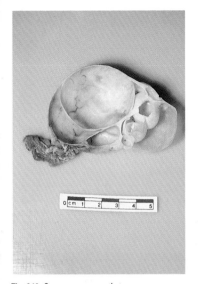

**Fig. 249** Ovary: serous cystic tumour.

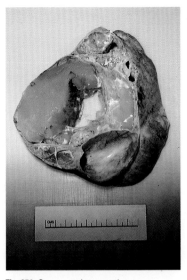

**Fig. 250** Ovary: mucinous cystic tumour.

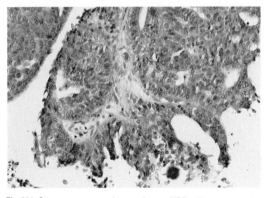

**Fig. 251** Ovary: serous cystadenocarcinoma. H&E ×25.

## Metastatic tumours

The ovary is a common site for metastases, especially from pelvic organs, breast and stomach. Krukenberg tumours are bilateral signet ring deposits usually from the stomach (Fig. 252).

## Sex cord stromal tumours

*Definition*  Neoplasms from sex cords of embryonal gonads.

*Incidence*  10% of ovarian tumours, mainly granulosa-theca tumours or fibromas. Sertoli-Leydig tumours are rare. Sex cord tumours may be hormonally active.

*Macroscopical*  Granulosa-theca tumours are yellow/orange solid or partly cystic encapsulated tumours. Fibromas are solid lobulated grey masses, while Sertoli-Leydig tumours often have foci of necrosis and haemorrhage.

*Microscopical*  Granulosa-theca tumours have granulosa cells in cords, sheets or glandular formation with acidophilic material (Call-Exner rosettes) (Fig. 253). Fibromas show spindle shaped fibroblasts with scanty collagenous tissue. Sertoli-Leydig tumours consist of normal cells growing in tubules or sarcomatous pattern.

*Prognosis*  Granulosa-theca tumours may produce oestrogen; about 10% of patients will develop endometrial carcinoma and 5–25% are malignant. Fibromas are benign but may be associated with pleural effusion and ascites (Meig's syndrome). 5% of Sertoli-Leydig tumours recur or metastasize.

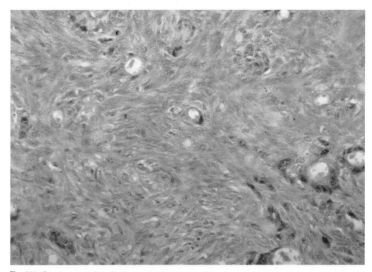

**Fig. 252** Ovary: metastatic gastric carcinoma (Kruckenburg tumour). H&E ×40.

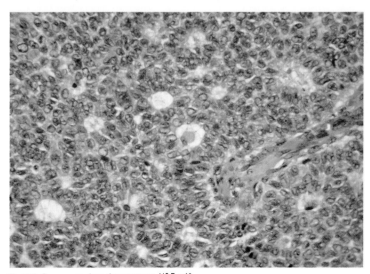

**Fig. 253** Ovary: granulosa-theca tumour. H&E ×40.

# Index